MAD STUDIES

THE BASICS

Mad Studies: The Basics provides an introductory account of a field that emerged from, and must remain grounded within, community knowledge, activism, and the perspectives of those who have experienced madness and mental health systems.

It is a concise text that introduces the field through an exploration of some origins of Mad Studies, as well as two interrelated queries: what does Mad Studies help us understand, and what does Mad Studies help us do? This exploration reveals that Mad Studies is an interdisciplinary, intersectional, and multi-vocal field that demands different answers to the very meaning of the beliefs, behaviours, and bodymind experiences that are currently characterized as being indicative of mental illness. At the heart of Mad Studies is a liberationist desire to resist, transform, and abolish the systems that create marginalization, and implement responses to madness that are grounded in the collective knowledge of those deemed Mad. This book shows that the contributions of Indigenous, Black, racialized, queer, and trans people must be understood as central to, and already embedded within, Mad Studies and activism rather than as add-ons, expansions, or efforts to make Mad Studies more inclusive.

It will be of interest to all scholars and students of disability studies, social work, gender studies, education, health sciences, sociology, and psychology, as well as practitioners in mental health care, and those with lived experience of madness and mental health systems.

Merrick Daniel Pilling is Assistant Professor in the School of Disability Studies at Toronto Metropolitan University. He is the author of *Queer and Trans Madness: Struggles for Social Justice* and co-editor of *Interrogating Psychiatric Narratives of Madness: Documented Lives*.

MAD STUDIES

THE BASICS

Merrick Daniel Pilling

Routledge
Taylor & Francis Group

LONDON AND NEW YORK

Designed cover image: Getty Image Number 1418278739

First published 2025
by Routledge
4 Park Square, Milton Park, Abingdon, Oxon OX14 4RN

and by Routledge
605 Third Avenue, New York, NY 10158

Routledge is an imprint of the Taylor & Francis Group, an informa business

© 2025 **Merrick Daniel Pilling**

British Library Cataloguing-in-Publication Data
A catalogue record for this book is available from the British Library

ISBN: 978-1-032-71988-7 (hbk)
ISBN: 978-1-032-91138-0 (pbk)
ISBN: 978-1-003-56155-2 (ebk)

DOI: 10.4324/9781003561552

Typeset in Sabon
by codeMantra

For all those deemed Mad; past, present, and future

CONTENTS

ACKNOWLEDGEMENTS

Thank you to all the activists and Mad people who brought Mad Studies into being; the impact of your work is incommensurable. Thanks are due to Tasha Sioufi Stansbury for her hard work on formatting the chapter reference lists. Thank you to Jijian Voronka for comments on the survivor research section of Chapter 3, and to the anonymous peer reviewers who provided helpful feedback on the book proposal and the manuscript. Thank you to my partner, Keith, I am so grateful for you.

INTRODUCTION – MAD STUDIES
The Basics

Mad Studies is intentionally slippery and indeterminate. It resists authoritative definition and remains dynamic, pluralistic, evolving, and collectively generated (Costa, 2014; Gorman & LeFrançois, 2017; LeFrançois et al., 2013). This book therefore does not attempt to define, own, or firmly outline the boundaries of the field. And yet, if Mad Studies is not everything, it must be something. This book provides a partial accounting of a field that emerged from, and must remain accountable to, community knowledge, activism, and the perspectives of those who have been psychiatrized and dehumanized by the psy complex and other exploitative systems of power.[1] It does so through an explanation of some origins of Mad Studies, and an exploration of two interrelated queries: what does Mad Studies help us understand, and what does Mad Studies help us do? This exploration reveals that Mad Studies is an interdisciplinary, intersectional, and multi-vocal field that demands different answers to the very meaning of the beliefs, behaviours, and bodymind experiences that are currently characterized as being indicative of mental illness. At the heart of Mad Studies is a liberationist desire to resist, transform, and abolish the systems that create marginalization, and implement frameworks

DOI: 10.4324/9781003561552-1

and responses to madness and distress that are grounded within the collective knowledge of those deemed Mad.

This book is written with post-secondary students in mind, to serve as an introduction to the growing field of Mad Studies. It will also be useful to anyone who wants a snapshot of the field, including practitioners in health care and social services, and those with lived experience of madness and mental health systems (these groups, of course, are not mutually exclusive). This book is also an exercise in field-building; as an area of study with several flagship texts and an international journal, it is high time for an introductory text to support the proliferation of Mad Studies and Mad pedagogy.

As a concise introduction to the field, this book only scratches the surface of what has been written on any given topic in Mad Studies. For each term, concept, and subject introduced, there is much more to be said. I hope this will spark interest in Mad Studies and inspire readers to read more deeply on the topics they find interesting. There may be those who disagree with my framing of Mad Studies, and what I have included and excluded. Indeed, there are those who disagree with the academicizing of Mad Studies who may balk at any attempt to crystallize the field and further entrench this knowledge within the academic industrial complex (Archibald, 2024; Ingram, 2016). Many questions and concerns haunt the establishment of Mad Studies within the academy. Will Mad Studies become co-opted by neoliberal forces, excluding the very people who brought its foundational concepts into existence? Will it stray too far from its radical roots in community activism, becoming politically and ethically bankrupt? Will Mad ideas and practices that cannot be co-opted be jettisoned, thereby smoothing out Mad Studies' abolitionist and radical edges to make it more palatable to the neoliberal university? Will relatively privileged Mad Studies scholars in academia erase the interests of those most heavily impacted by forces of marginalization? Will Mad Studies become a largely inaccessible theoretical exercise, casting aside political action and the 'doing' of Mad resistance? In writing this book aimed at bringing Mad Studies to a wider audience, am I ushering in such horrors? These are legitimate concerns. Critical ideas and practices can easily be perverted to serve the interests of neoliberal institutions, services, and governments. We have already witnessed the co-option of core contributions of Mad activists and scholars such as the concept of recovery, the practice of peer support, and even narratives of lived experience (Beresford, 2019; Beresford & Russo, 2016; Costa et al., 2012; Fabris, 2013; Joseph, 2019; Pilling, 2019; Voronka, 2017, 2019a, 2019b). And yet, I believe that Mad Studies has the potential to continue to disrupt, challenge, subvert, and resist exploitative power relations and the systems that create marginalization. I also believe Mad Studies can continue to honour and reclaim survivor narratives, experiences, and ways of being and knowing, and restore dignity and collective care to those who have been psychiatrized, criminalized, and dehumanized.

My hope is that this book will introduce Mad Studies to a broad range of diversely situated students, academics, people with lived experience, and those in direct service who will use this knowledge to support and radicalize the work they do in the world. I hope that it will be used as a teaching tool to disrupt the perspectives within which we are all steeped that position madness as mental illness, and challenge educational practices within the psydisciplines and other fields that currently oppress Mad people through the imposition of biomedical frameworks (i.e. Social Work, Nursing, Psychology, Psychiatry, and beyond). I believe there are many academics, practitioners, and people with lived experience who know that something is wrong with the way people are treated within mental health systems and feel like something is missing from what they have been taught in school or at work about mental illness who would welcome the perspectives that Mad Studies provides. This includes Mad people; whether Mad or not, we have all been immersed in the biomedical model because it is constructed as 'common sense,' and Mad Studies perspectives are not widely available. I hope this book will be a tool for understanding how Mad Studies allows us to see the personal, the political, and the theoretical differently when it comes to experiences of, and responses to, madness and distress.

This book, and Mad Studies as a whole, must be mindful of resisting white-centric and cishetero-centric genealogies and accountings of the field. Other social justice-based academic fields and their associated social movements such as Disability Studies and the disability rights movement and Women's Studies and the feminist movement have been justly critiqued for favouring the relatively privileged among the marginalized, thereby upholding white supremacy and cisheteropatriarchy. Mad Studies is relatively young, and critiques of white supremacy and the necessity of attending to the experiences of racialized and Indigenous people were expressed early in the development of Mad Studies as an academic field (Gorman, 2013; Gorman et al., 2013; Jackson, 2002; Kalathil, 2013; Kanani, 2011; Tam, 2013). It is important to emphasize that analyses of racism and the labour of Indigenous and racialized people have always been present and integral to the formation of the field, even while the pressures of white supremacy attempt to elide and marginalize this work while uplifting white scholars and activists (Gorman & LeFrançois, 2017). That said, erasures persist, and the articulation of intersectional, decolonial, and anti-racist analyses, histories, and practices is necessary and ongoing (Costa & Ross, 2023; Dwornik, 2021; Kalathil & Jones, 2016; Joseph, 2015, 2019; Lavallée & Poole, 2010; Redikopp, 2021). Likewise, Mad Studies (and therefore this book) is dominated by Global North perspectives and issues, though there are exceptions and recent shifts in this regard (Davar, 2021; Nabbali, 2013; Eromosele, 2022; Persaud, 2022; Sharma, 2022, 2023). More specifically, given my own location, many of the examples used throughout this book are Canadian.

Readers may also notice that explorations of the intersections between madness and cisheteronormativity are not as prominent as they should be in the field of Mad Studies. Explorations of the mutually constitutive nature of cisheteronormativity and sanism have not been featured prominently in Mad Studies, despite the obvious overlaps between Queer Studies, Trans Studies, and Mad Studies and their respective associated activist struggles for social justice (Cosantino & Pilling, 2024;

Diamond, 2017; LeFrançois & Diamond, 2014; Pilling, 2022, forthcoming; Spandler & Barker, 2016) and the long history and ongoing practice of psychiatric violence against trans, non-binary, and queer people (Pilling, 2022, forthcoming). Certainly, there are queer and trans voices in Mad Studies, however, there is room to pursue more avenues of inquiry given that notions of sanity are built upon requirements of cisgenderism and gender normativity (Daley, 2021; Pilling, 2022, forthcoming). This is all the more important because of the recent rise in transphobic violence across many nation-states (both state violence and interpersonal violence) and the way such violence is often expressed through intersections of transphobia with sanism, ableism, and other forms of oppression.

LANGUAGE AND TERMINOLOGY

The language we use matters. The words we choose are not neutral; they betray underlying ideologies and reveal something about what is believed to be true about the topic at hand. Through the words we use, we can uphold or resist dominant discourses and prevailing ways of thinking. For example, Mad Studies scholars have been justly critiqued for using colonialism as an analogy for psychiatric domination, thereby dismissing those who have experienced both colonization and psychiatric domination and eliding the ways in which psychiatry is inextricably bound up with colonialism (Gorman et al., 2013; Mills, 2017). As Gorman et al. (2013) state, "white people's experiences of psychiatry are not 'like colonialism.' Colonialism is like colonialism" (para. 11).

Throughout this book I am purposeful about the language I use. I employ the term 'Mad' in various ways, but mainly as an umbrella term to indicate a politicized way of thinking and doing that is different from research and services aimed at addressing 'mental health' and 'mental illness,' which are terms that belong to "an entirely different discourse" (Burstow, 2013, p. 79). Previously used to denigrate, 'Mad' has been reclaimed by some as an identity as well as a theoretical concept and descriptor (e.g. Mad Studies, Mad pedagogy, Mad praxis, Mad activism, etc.). At times I use 'Mad' or 'madness' to denote behaviours that transgress social norms and the prevailing social order, beliefs that stray from those that are commonly accepted within society, and bodymind experiences that are positioned as abnormal, undesirable, or bizarre. This use of 'Mad' and 'madness' should not be conflated with self-identification, since such behaviours, beliefs, and experiences can be positioned as madness *whether or not* the person or group attached to them self-identify as Mad. In some places I use 'Mad' as a non-essentialized identity category, while recognizing that this term cannot be seen as being inclusive of all those who have been oppressed by the psy complex and other systems of marginalization. As explained in more detail in Chapter 2, the term is limited when it comes to the recognition of the experiences of Indigenous, Black, racialized, and two-spirit, lesbian, gay, bisexual, trans, queer, and intersex (2SLGBTQI) people.

WHO AM I, TO WRITE THIS BOOK?

I do not position myself as 'the expert' on Mad Studies. Rather, I offer a critical summary of some parts of this rapidly expanding field as I see it (and participate in it) from my necessarily biased perspective. I have written elsewhere about some of my personal attachments to Mad Studies (Pilling, 2022). It shaped my graduate education and continues to be a large part of my ongoing academic career as a professor in a School of Disability Studies. Perhaps more importantly, I see the ethos of collective care embedded in Mad Studies as potentially lifesaving. I am eager to see a proliferation of resistance and alternatives to coercive and carceral 'treatment' (such as those outlined in Chapter 3) because I believe it can save the lives of my friends, family, students, colleagues, and community members both known and unknown to me. I hope that this book can support and contribute to these efforts by bringing Mad Studies to a wider audience and by continuing to build the field.

CHAPTER SUMMARIES

CHAPTER 1: SOME ORIGINS OF MAD STUDIES

The ideas, concepts, and practices that inform Mad Studies have existed in community and grassroots activism for much longer than Mad Studies has been recognized as an academic field of study. Chapter 1 is a partial exploration of how Mad Studies came to be, examining some of the origins of Mad Studies while arguing that these are multiple, intersecting, and incomplete. This chapter cautions against the whitewashing and cis-heterosexualizing of the origins of Mad Studies and briefly outlines some its roots in the Mad movement, Black Power, Gay Liberation, and trans activism. Finally, this chapter traces the emergence of Mad Studies within academia and its relationship to overlapping fields such as Disability Studies and Gender and Women's Studies.

CHAPTER 2: WHAT CAN MAD STUDIES HELP US UNDERSTAND?

Chapter 2 explores some answers to the question, what can Mad Studies help us understand? Rather than providing an authoritative definition of Mad Studies, this chapter discusses some of the key concepts, frameworks, and areas of study that Mad Studies can help us understand. It is explained how Mad Studies explicates the biomedical model of mental illness as the prevailing framework for understanding and responding to madness and distress and how this framework is connected to the larger psy complex. Various ways of conceptualizing madness and distress within Mad Studies are explored, including the use of the social/biological binary to make sense of madness. The Mad Studies concept of bodymind is then used to highlight some of the problems with binary frameworks and demonstrate the uses of non-binary theorizing about madness. Chapter 2 also includes a discussion of the value and pitfalls of Mad as an identity, as well as a section on sanism and epistemic injustice. The chapter concludes with an exploration of the use of a Mad lens to examine the process of knowledge production. This final section demonstrates how Mad Studies can help us reexamine who produces knowledge and how, with whose interests in mind, and with whose bodies on the line.

CHAPTER 3: WHAT CAN MAD STUDIES HELP US DO?

Originating as it does in community activism, Mad Studies is action-oriented and can provide some tools for doing things differently. Following Costa and Ross (2023), the premise of Chapter 3 is that "Mad Studies... is itself praxis" (p. 4). The chapter begins with an exploration of the praxis-oriented aspects of employing a Mad lens, including the use of madness as an analytic, that is, to 'madden.' The rest of the chapter focuses on various other aspects of Mad praxis, or in other words, putting Mad Studies into action. This includes a section on survivor research, showing how notions of expertise have been reclaimed by those with experiential knowledge who are working towards epistemic justice. It also includes a section on Mad pedagogy, and another on Mad art as praxis. The final section covers how Mad people resist psychiatric violence, including though creating different approaches to care and treatment. This includes a discussion of resistance to coercive care and electroconvulsive therapy (ECT), and an exploration of the Mad practice of peer support and its struggles with co-option.

Recommended resources

Costa, L. & Ross, L. (2023). Mad Studies genealogy and praxis. *International Mad Studies Journal*, 1(1), e1–8. https://doi.org/10.58544/imsj.v1i1.5239

Gorman, R., saini, a., Tam, L., Udegbe, O., & Usar, O. (2013). Mad people of colour: A manifesto. *Asylum*, 20(4), 27. https://asylummagazine.org/2013/12/mad-people-of-color-a-manifesto-by-rachel-gorman-annu-saini-louise-tam-onyinyechukwu-udegbe-onar-usar/

Madness Network News. (n.d.). *Definitions*. https://madnessnetworknews.com/definitions/

Spandler, H., & Barker M.-J. (2016, July 1). *Mad and queer studies: Interconnections and tensions*. Mad Studies Network. https://madstudies2014.wordpress.com/2016/07/01/mad-and-queer-studies-interconnections-and-tensions/

NOTE

1 For those unfamiliar with the term 'psychiatrized' and other such terms used throughout this book, please consult Madness Network News' comprehensive list of collectively created definitions: https://madnessnetworknews.com/definitions/

REFERENCES

Archibald, L. (2024). Maintaining the fidelity of Mad Studies (An ode to Mad Studies 2). *Asylum, 31*(1), 16–17.

Beresford, P. (2019). Including our self in struggle: Challenging the neo-liberal psycho-system's subversion of us, our ideas and action. *Canadian Journal of Disability Studies, 8*(4), 31–59. https://doi.org/10.15353/cjds.v8i4.523

Beresford, P. & Russo, J. (2016). Supporting the sustainability of Mad Studies and preventing its co-option. *Disability & Society, 31*(2), 270–274. https://doi.org/10.1080/09687599.2016.1145380

Burstow, B. (2013). A rose by any other name: Naming and the battle against psychiatry. In B. A. LeFrançois, R. Menzies, & G. Reaume (Eds.), *Mad matters: A critical reader in Canadian Mad Studies* (pp. 79–90). Canadian Scholars Press.

Cosantino, J. & Pilling, M. (2024, September 7). *Forging a MadTrans Studies* [Conference presentation]. The 2nd International Trans Studies Conference, Northwestern University, Evanston, IL, United States.

Costa, L. (2014, October 15). *Mad Studies – What it is and why you should care*. Mad Studies Network. https://mad-studies2014.wordpress.com/2014/10/15/mad-studies-what-it-is-and-why-you-should-care-2/

Costa, L. & Ross, L. (2023). Mad Studies genealogy and praxis. *International Mad Studies Journal, 1*(1), e1–8. https://doi.org/10.58544/imsj.v1i1.5239

Costa, L., Voronka, J., Landry, D., Reid, J., Mcfarlane, B., Reville, D., & Church, K. (2012). "Recovering our stories": A small act of resistance. *Studies in Social Justice, 6*(1), 85–101. https://doi.org/10.26522/ssj.v6i1.1070

Daley, A. (2021). Narrating genders in psychiatric inpatient chart documentation. In A. Daley & M. D. Pilling (Eds.), *Interrogating psychiatric narratives of madness: Documented lives* (pp. 57–86). Palgrave MacMillan. https://doi.org/10.1007/978-3-030-83692-4_3

Davar, B. V. (2021). Shifting identities as reflective personal responses to political changes. In P. Beresford and J. Russo (Eds.), *The Routledge international handbook of Mad Studies* (pp. 34–40). Routledge. https://doi.org/10.4324/9780429465444-5

Diamond, S. (2017). Trapped in change: Using queer theory to examine the progress of psy-theories and interventions with sexuality and gender. In B. M. Z. Cohen (Ed.), *Routledge international handbook of critical mental health* (pp. 89–97). Routledge. https://doi.org/10.4324/9781315399584-12

Dwornik, A. (2021). The interface of Mad Studies and Indigenous ways of knowing: Innovation, co-creation, and decolonization. *Critical Social Work*, *22*(2), 24–39. https://doi.org/10.22329/csw.v22i2.7097

Eromosele, F. (2022). Madness, decolonization and mental health activism in Africa. In P. Beresford and J. Russo (Eds.), *The Routledge international handbook of Mad Studies* (pp. 327–339). Routledge. https://doi.org/10.4324/9780429465444-38

Fabris, E. (2013). Mad success: What could go wrong when psychiatry employs us as "peers"? In B. A. LeFrançois, R. Menzies, & G. Reaume (Eds.), *Mad matters: A critical reader in Canadian Mad Studies* (pp. 130–139). Canadian Scholars Press.

Gorman, R. (2013). Thinking through race, class, and mad identity politics. In B. A. LeFrançois, R. Menzies, & G. Reaume (Eds.), *Mad matters: A critical reader in Canadian Mad Studies* (pp. 269–280). Canadian Scholars Press.

Gorman, R., saini, a., Tam, L., Udegbe, O., & Usar, O. (2013). Mad people of colour: A manifesto. *Asylum*, *20*(4), 27. https://asylummagazine.org/2013/12/mad-people-of-color-a-manifesto-by-rachel-gorman-annu-saini-louise-tam-onyinyechukwu-udegbe-onar-usar/

Gorman, R. & Lefrançois, B. A. (2017). Mad Studies. In B. M. Z. Cohen (Ed.), *Routledge international handbook of critical mental health* (pp. 107–114). Routledge. https://doi. org/10.4324/9781315399584-14

Ingram, R. A. (2016). Doing mad studies: Making (non)sense together. *Intersectionalities: A Global Journal of Social Work Analysis, Research, Polity, and Practice, 5*(3), 11–17.

Jackson, V. (2002). In our own voice: African-American stories of oppression, survival and recovery in mental health systems. *International Journal of Narrative Therapy and Community Work, 2,* 11–31.

Joseph, A. J. (2015). The necessity of an attention to Euro-centrism and colonial technologies: An addition to critical mental health literature. *Disability & Society, 30*(7), 1021–1041. https://doi.org/10.1080/09687599.2015.1067187

Joseph, A. J. (2019). Constituting "lived experience" discourses in mental health: The ethics of racialized identification/ representation and the erasure of intergeneration colonial violence. *Journal of Ethics in Mental Health, 10,* 1–23.

Kalathil, J. (2013). "Hard to reach"? Racialized groups and mental health service user involvement. In P. Staddon (Ed.), *Mental health service users in research: Critical sociological perspectives* (pp. 121–133). Policy Press. https://doi. org/10.1332/policypress/9781447307334.003.0009

Kalathil, J. & Jones, N. (2016). Unsettling disciplines: Madness, identity, research, knowledge. *Philosophy, Psychiatry, & Psychology, 23*(3), 183–188. https://doi.org/10.1353/ ppp.2016.0016

Kanani, N. (2011). Race and madness: Locating the experiences of racialized people with psychiatric histories in Canada and the United States. *Critical Disability Discourse, 3,* 1–14.

Lavallée, L. F. & Poole, J. M. (2010). Beyond recovery: Colonization, health and healing for Indigenous people in Canada. *International Journal of Mental Health and Addiction, 8,* 271–281.

Lefrançois, B. A. & Diamond, S. (2014). Queering the sociology of diagnosis: Children and the constituting of "mentally ill" subjects. *Journal of Critical Anti-Oppressive Social Inquiry*, *1*(1), 39–61.

LeFrançois, B. A., Menzies, R., & Reaume, G. (Eds.). (2013). *Mad matters: A critical reader in Canadian Mad Studies*. Canadian Scholars Press.

Madness Network News. (n.d.). *Definitions*. https://madness-networknews.com/definitions/

Mills, C. (2017). Global psychiatrization and psychic colonization: The coloniality of global mental health. In M. Morrow and L. Malcoe (Eds.), *Critical inquiries for social justice in mental health* (pp. 87–109). University of Toronto Press. https://doi.org/10.3138/9781442619708-005

Nabbali, E. M. (2013). "Mad" activism and its (Ghanaian?) future: A prolegomena to debate. *Trans-Scripts*, *3*, 178–201.

Persaud, S. (2022). *No sovereign remedy: Distress, madness, and mental health care in Guyana* [Doctoral dissertation, York University]. YorkSpace.

Pilling, M. D. (2019). Changing directions or staying the course? Recovery, gender, and sexuality in Canada's mental health strategy. In A. Daley, L. Costa, & P. Beresford (Eds.), *Madness, violence, and power: A critical collection* (pp. 97–114). University of Toronto Press. https://doi.org/10.3138/9781442629981-012

Pilling, M. D. (2022). *Queer and trans madness: Struggles for social justice*. Palgrave MacMillan.

Pilling, M. D. (Forthcoming). Toward mad trans liberation: The necessity of a mad-queer-trans lens. In B. LeFrançois, I. Abdillahi, G. Reaume, & R. Menzies (Eds.), *Mad matters: A critical reader in Canadian Mad Studies* (2nd ed.). Canadian Scholars Press.

Redikopp, S. (2021). Out of place, out of mind: Min(d)ing race in Mad Studies through a metaphor of spatiality. *Canadian Journal of Disability Studies*, *10*(3), 96–118. https://doi.org/10.15353/cjds.v10i3.817

Sharma, P. (2022). Navigating voices, politics, positions amidst peers: Resonances and dissonances in India. In P. Beresford and J. Russo (Eds.), *The Routledge international handbook* of *Mad Studies* (pp. 340–350). Routledge. https://doi.org/10.4324/9780429465444-39

Sharma, P. (2023). *Barriers to recovery from "psychosis": A peer investigation of psychiatric subjectivation.* Routledge. https://doi.org/10.4324/9781003248804

Spandler, H. & Barker M.-J. (2016, July 1). *Mad and queer studies: Interconnections and tensions.* Mad Studies Network. https://madstudies2014.wordpress.com/2016/07/01/mad-and-queer-studies-interconnections-and-tensions/

Tam, L. (2013). Whither indigenizing the mad movement? Theorizing the social relations of race and madness through conviviality. In B. A. LeFrançois, R. Menzies, & G. Reaume (Eds.), *Mad matters: A critical reader in Canadian Mad Studies* (pp. 281–297). Canadian Scholars Press.

Voronka, J. (2017). Turning mad knowledge into affective labor: The case of the peer support worker. *American Quarterly*, 69(2), 333–338. https://doi.org/10.1353/aq.2017.0029

Voronka, J. (2019a). Storytelling beyond the psychiatric gaze: Resisting resilience and recovery narratives. *Canadian Journal of Disability Studies*, 8(4), 8–30. https://doi.org/10.15353/cjds.v8i4.522

Voronka, J. (2019b). The mental health peer worker as informant: Performing authenticity and the paradoxes of passing. *Disability & Society*, 34(4), 564–582. https://doi.org/10.1080/09687599.2018.1545113

SOME ORIGINS OF MAD STUDIES

There is no single truth about the creation of Mad Studies and no origin story should be taken up as rigid, fixed, exhaustive, or as the most authentic version. The title of this chapter uses the phrase '*some* origins' instead of '*the* origins' of Mad Studies to signal that there are many different stories that could be told about how Mad Studies came to be, and there are multiple locations from which it can be said to have arisen. One thing that is certain is that the ideas, concepts, and practices that inform Mad Studies have existed in communities and grass-roots activism for much longer than the creation of Mad Studies as an academic field, which was named as such in the early 2000s. The majority of this chapter is devoted to exploring some of these activist roots of Mad Studies in the Mad move-ment of the 1970s in Canada and the United States, as well as in other social justice movements of the same era, such as Black Power, Gay Liberation, and trans activism.[1] The remain-der of the chapter focuses on the emergence of Mad Studies in academia and its relationship to overlapping fields such as Disability Studies and Gender and Women's Studies.

There are many theorists whose work predates the naming of Mad Studies, but whom some claim as influential in the

DOI: 10.4324/9781003561552-2

development of Mad Studies, such as Frantz Fanon and Michel Foucault. However, the purpose of this chapter is to point to some of the origins of Mad Studies in community organizing and various bodies of knowledge rather than to delve into the ideas of any one theorist or activist. As Menzies et al. (2013) state, Mad Studies is "a loose assemblage of perspectives that resist compression into an irreducible dogma or singular approach to theory or practice" (p. 13). This chapter will point to precursors of some of the vectors within that 'loose assemblage' while acknowledging that there are many others, and that these will vary across local contexts. The primary focus is on the 1960s onwards, but it is possible to look further back in history for some origins of Mad Studies (see for example Reaume, 2024) though there are challenges in doing so when it comes to Indigenous, Black, and racialized people's perspectives.

RESISTING THE WHITEWASHING AND CIS-HETEROSEXUALIZING OF MAD STUDIES ORIGINS

It is essential to resist the whitewashing and cis-heterosexualizing of Mad Studies by locating its roots primarily in the activism and scholarship of white, cisgender, heterosexual people.[2] The contributions of Indigenous, Black, racialized, queer, and trans people must be understood as central to, and already embedded within, Mad Studies and Mad activism rather than as add-ons, expansions, or efforts to make Mad Studies more inclusive. As will be further discussed in Chapters 2 and 3, conceptualizations of sanity and reason rely upon normative ideals of gender and sexuality (Daley, 2021; Hectors, 2023; Pilling, 2022). Likewise, notions of reason and rationality have long been used to demarcate Indigenous, Black, and racialized people as incapable of reason and as primitive, uncivilized, and biologically inferior (Bruce, 2021; Fernando, 2010). Constructs of insanity and feeblemindedness have been mobilized against Indigenous, Black, and racialized people in the service of land theft and white nation building (Joseph, 2014, 2019).

Any exploration of madness and sanism must therefore engage with colonialism, anti-Blackness, and cisheteronormativity as mutually constitutive systems of power, and centre the resistance of Black, Indigenous, racialized, queer, and trans people. This requires deliberate and creative efforts to unearth these histories of resistance because of their suppression and erasure. Writing of his great-grandmother, Joseph (2022) recounts that she was born on a boat transporting indentured labourers from Calcutta to Guyana and was identified on her son's birth certificate by the name of this boat and a registration number rather than by her last name. Joseph states that "Her history is actively suppressed by the technologies of eradication that actively authorized dehumanization for the specific purposes of colonial nation building and exploitation" (p. 138). Joseph's account illustrates the power relations at play in suppressing individual and collective histories of racialized peoples, which suggests that there are also specific challenges in preserving and accounting for personal and collective histories of resistance. As Jackson (2002) explains, such histories of resistance are often not recorded, and white dominance within activist movements creates and compounds these erasures:

> There were thousands of African-American activists who resisted psychiatric oppression on a daily basis, but many of them are lost to us because they are not recorded in the official history. We can no longer wait for the predominately white consumer/survivors/ex-patients movement to include us as an addendum to their history. We will have to write our own history to celebrate our legacy of resistance.
>
> (p. 18)

As this also suggests, histories of Black people's resistance are already embedded in Mad Studies and activism even if they have not been recorded. It is important not to conflate *suppression and erasure* with *absence* because doing so reifies the erasure of Indigenous, Black, and racialized people's resistance.

In addition to the suppression and erasure of Indigenous, Black, and racialized people's histories of Mad resistance, the language and approaches used may be different from mainstream activist efforts and therefore may not be recognized by some as Mad resistance (Lavallée, 2021; Schalk, 2022). For example, Schalk (2022) argues that Black activist approaches to madness and disability are "intersectional but race centered, not (necessarily) based in disability identity, contextualized and historicized, and holistic" (p. 12). As will be discussed further in Chapter 2, a Mad identity may not appeal in the same way to Indigenous, Black, racialized, queer, and trans communities. This means that activist efforts and resistance to psychiatric oppression by these groups might not always use the language of madness. As Schalk's (2022) work indicates, approaches that are intersectional in nature or that centre other systemic power relations such as racism (rather than *only* sanism or ableism) may not be recognized as Mad activism because they operate differently than the single-issue politics that tend to dominate mainstream (white-centric) activism. Pickens' (2019) work shows that this is also the case when it comes to examining literature and scholarly works. Pickens argues that discussions of disability, madness, and Blackness may use different language and citational practices and thus may result in the mistaken assumption that a discussion of race and disability is absent:

> when Blackness and disability cohere, they challenge each other institutionally and allow for the possibility that disability or race may be called by other names. As with the language of madness, no language regarding disability is neutral, which means that the euphemisms in common parlance ... make their way into critical literature differently as well ... What appears to be a gap in this discussion of race and disability actually requires a rereading of the critical literature, since in Black cultural and critical contexts, disability is often operating in other registers ... one has to think Blackly or madly.
>
> (pp. 8–9)

I understand Pickens' work as a reminder to pay attention to what is already there, and that when looking for Black Mad resistance another lens and way of reading and understanding will be necessary. In addition to thinking 'Blackly or madly,' other strategies may be helpful in centering and unearthing Indigenous, Black, and racialized people's Mad resistance. Methods include reading against the grain of institutional records of asylums and hospitals to unearth examples of Indigenous, Black, and racialized people's resistance to the psy complex (see for example Hylton, 2024; Walker, 2022). Jackson (2002) suggests that conducting oral histories with Black psychiatric survivors is a way of "restorying" Black lives and histories of resistance (p. 13). She also proposes examining narratives of those who were enslaved to glean information about how those who were deemed insane were treated and how they dealt with distress (Jackson, 2002, p. 27). These methods are invaluable and yet are also limited in terms of their time span as they cannot address the days that predate written institutional records, and institutional records do not capture first-person accounts. However, it is crucial that Mad Studies refuses to reify the erasure of Indigenous, Black, and racialized people's Mad resistance by acting as if it did not happen because there are no written records of it. Indigenous peoples who were dispossessed of their lands, Black people who were enslaved, and other racialized peoples who were exploited in the name of nation building were the furthest from benefitting from the status quo and therefore had the deepest insight into exploitative power relations, and no doubt resisted the way they were positioned and treated. While we do not have historical records of first-person accounts of what could be called Mad resistance that date as far back as those of white wealthy people, we can be confident that such resistance took place.

Conducting primary research is beyond the scope of this book, and thus this chapter relies on what has already been written about histories of Mad resistance in order to create multiple narratives about some of the origins of Mad Studies. There are therefore some limitations in terms of what is included about the resistance of Indigenous, Black, and racialized people, given that much of what has been written about the Mad movement has been by and about white activists even though Mad people of colour have always been active participants and organizers (Landry, 2023). To broaden the scope of what is included and to continue the conversation about how the Mad resistance of queer, trans, Indigenous, Black, and racialized people may look different outside of white, heterosexual spaces, I draw on writings about Black Power, Gay Liberation, and trans activism instead of focusing only on what has been written about the Mad movement. As Landry (2023) points out, much of the history of Indigenous, Black, and racialized people's Mad resistance "remains tucked away in personal archives: in boxes, scrapbooks and photo albums, in need of preserving" (p. 775). As she goes on to argue, community archives such as Madness Canada's (madnesscanada.com/resources/archives) can "rectify historical erasures" (p. 775). I am hopeful that the future will see more documentation and digital preservation of personal archives that detail the Mad resistance of queer, trans, Indigenous, Black, and racialized people.

THE MAD MOVEMENT

The Mad movement in Canada and the United States arose in the 1970s in the context of other intersecting social movements of the time such as feminism, Black Power, Gay Liberation, and disability rights, though it has often been excluded from histories of social movements (Beckman & Davies, 2013). Currently, it is frequently referred to as the Mad movement (or movements), but it also goes by other names. These include the psychiatric survivor movement, mental patients' liberation movement, consumer/survivor/ex-patient (c/s/x) movement, Mad pride movement, and the service user/survivor movement, amongst others. These various names reflect the local contexts within which they are used, as well as the fact that the movement has always been multi-vocal. The name c/s/x is perhaps the most illustrative of this, as the three terms (consumer, survivor, and ex-patient) reflect varying ideologies and relationships to psychiatry and the mental health system.

The term 'consumer' can be seen as emphasizing choice in the 'marketplace' of health services, while 'ex-patient' and 'survivor' can be seen as critical of psychiatry as a form of violence that has been survived (for a more detailed discussion of terminology see Reaume, 2002). The movement has always included those with an abolitionist stance as well as those who seek reform and cooperation with mental health services and in fact have often "met in the middle"[3] (Morrison, 2005, p. 57).

The Mad movement is not the same thing as the anti-psychiatry movement, though it is frequently misunderstood and mislabelled as such. Arising in the 1960s, the anti-psychiatry movement was led by mainly white men academics and mental health professionals (e.g. psychiatrists and psychologists) who had become disenchanted with some aspects of their profession and, to varying degrees, critiqued the biomedical model of mental illness and argued against coerced treatment (Chamberlin, 1990; Reaume, 2022). Thinkers such as David Cooper, R. D. Laing, Thomas Szasz, Erving Goffman, and Michel Foucault have all been called anti-psychiatry, though many were not self-described as such (Reaume, 2022). The anti-psychiatry movement is often characterized as academic and elitist because there was little effort made to connect with Mad community or to include the perspectives of those with lived experience of mental health systems (Reaume, 2022). While the Mad movement was influenced by anti-psychiatry (among other ways of thinking) and some Mad activists (past and present) also identify as anti-psychiatry, the Mad movement should not be conflated with the anti-psychiatry movement.[4]

The Mad movement of the 1970s was comprised of small, independent, local collectives created and led by people who had experienced mental health systems. The first Canadian collective, the Mental Patients Association (MPA) was created in 1971 in Vancouver, British Columbia by Lanny Beckman (Beckman & Davies, 2013). The group offered peer support, a drop-in centre, and eventually purchased housing for its members and set up a legal advocacy program (MPA Documentary Collective, 2013). The group used principles of participatory democracy to make all decisions, meaning that they used a non-hierarchical structure where everyone had an equal vote (Beckman & Davies, 2013; MPA Documentary Collective, 2013). The group created *In a Nutshell*, a publication by and for Mad people that included first-person perspectives, news, art, poetry, and more. The publication had subscribers across Canada and the U.S., and the MPA mailed copies to libraries around the world to increase circulation (MPA Documentary Collective, 2013). The MPA inspired others to create similar collectives. For example, in 1977, Don Weitz and Alf Jackson were inspired by MPA to create Ontario's Mental Patients Association (MPA), later renamed On Our Own (Reville & Church, 2012; Shimrat, 2018). In the words of Don Weitz, this group

> helped survivors re-develop social, practical and vocational skills that they had lost through psychiatric oppression. Our democratically run drop-in was a place of safety and empowerment, and our newsletter provided an outlet for the commentary and creativity that had been stifled by the 'mental health' system.
> (Weitz quoted in Shimrat, 2018)

In 1980, some of the members of Ontario's MPA created *Phoenix Rising: The Voice of the Psychiatrized*, a publication by and for psychiatric survivors that included first-person experiences, news, information about legal rights, art and poetry. It addressed issues of poverty, employment, discrimination, housing, and prisoners' rights, amongst other issues (Shimrat, 2018).

Similarly, local groups arose across the United States, beginning on the East and West coasts. These included the Insane Liberation Front in Portland in 1970, the Mental Patients' Liberation Project in New York City in 1971, and the Mental Patients' Liberation Front in Boston in 1971, amongst others (Chamberlin, 1990). These groups focused on self-help and advocacy, including advocating for people who were hospitalized, fighting for changes in laws regarding forced treatment, and performing direct actions at hospitals (Chamberlin, 1990).

In 1972, the San Francisco-based publication *Madness Network News* was created to report on the movement and like *In a Nutshell* and *Phoenix Rising: The Voice of the Psychiatrized*, it included first person accounts, art, creative writing, news, and political analyses of issues relevant to psychiatric survivors (Chamberlin, 1990; Lewis, 2006).[5] Beginning in 1973, the Conference on Human Rights and Psychiatric Oppression was held annually until 1985 as a way to bring together Mad advocates across the United States and Canada. These conferences provided an opportunity to network and share strategies and experiences (Chamberlin, 1990; Lewis, 2006). While the U.S.-based collectives and conference began with a mixed group of participants that included psychiatric survivors and mental health professionals, they eventually limited participation to those with lived experience because the involvement of professionals tended to blunt the radical edge of the collectives' politics (Chamberlin, 1990).

Popularized by Toronto-based Mad activist David Reville, the saying 'a home, a job, and a friend' summarizes some of the key foci of the Mad movement including the right to decent housing and employment, and combatting social isolation (Reville & Church, 2012). Further, the Mad movement was a place where Mad people began to speak for themselves rather than being spoken for, and assert the value of their own knowledge based on lived experience (Adame et al., 2017; Morrison, 2005). Psychiatric survivors sought access to information controlled by professionals, fought for more control over treatment, and to expose and put an end to psychiatric abuses (Morrison, 2005). The movement challenged psychiatric notions of lifelong disease with no cure and focused on creating peer-run alternatives that supported recovery from sanism, oppression, and abuse in mental health systems, rather than from mental illness (Howell & Voronka, 2012; Poole, 2011). Gathering with other survivors provided opportunities to challenge negative views of Mad people, both internal and external. As discussed below, for some, this evolved into a sense of Mad pride. The movement also sought to empower

Mad people to shift inequitable power relations and to recognize that individual experiences of psychiatric abuse and oppression are shared because they are systemic in nature and require collective action to create sustained change (Morrison, 2005). Groups across Canada and the U.S. fought to end coerced treatment, electroshock, and other abuses within mental health systems in their local contexts. Strategies employed include consciousness raising groups, self-help and peer support, drop-ins and skill building, direct actions such as protests, court challenges, participating in electoral politics and mayoral task forces, challenging zoning bylaws, creating social enterprises to employ Mad people, and creating conferences and publications (Adame et al., 2017; Beckman & Davies, 2013; Chamberlin, 1990; Lewis, 2006; Morrison, 2005; Reville & Church, 2012; Reaume, 2021; Starkman, 2013; Weitz, 2018).

Keeping in mind that this was before the days of the Internet, the importance of conferences and publications like *In a Nutshell*, *Phoenix Rising: The Voice of the Psychiatrized*, and *Madness Network News* cannot be overstated in terms of sharing information and linking local groups to the wider context of domestic and international Mad movements. Likewise, anthologies such as Burstow and Weitz's (1988*) Shrink Resistant: The Struggle Against Psychiatry in Canada*, and later, Shimrat's (1997) *Call me Crazy: Stories From the Mad Movement*, documented first-person accounts of the movement and are examples of creating knowledge and histories from a Mad perspective. In the U.S., Judi Chamberlin's (1978) *On our own: Patient Controlled Alternatives to the Mental Health System* was key in documenting and sharing Mad knowledge about creating alternatives by and for Mad people.

Mad movement groups operated with little to no funding and mostly ran on volunteer labour. Over time some of these collectives became more established and acquired funding, while others became defunct. Those like the Vancouver-based MPA who acquired funding became less radical as hierarchical organizational structures were imposed (MPA Documentary Collective, 2013). Key ideas from the broader Mad movement such as recovery have been co-opted and perverted by mainstream mental health systems to extend their reach and reassert their authority and expertise (Howell & Voronka, 2012; Poole, 2011; Voronka, 2019). However, elements of the radical ideas[6] of the 1970s and 1980s Mad movement collectives were carried into Mad organizing of the 1990s and into today, in the form of both Mad activism and Mad Studies.

PSYCHIATRIC SURVIVOR PRIDE DAY/MAD PRIDE

The first Psychiatric Survivor Pride Day (renamed Mad Pride in 2002) was created in Toronto in 1993 by a group of psychiatric survivors led by Chava Finkler, a psychiatric survivor who worked at Parkdale Community Legal Services. Finkler was inspired by gay and lesbian Pride as well as notions of pride within disability activism and Black community organizing (Finkler, 1997). The goals of the Pride events were to change the negative public and self-image of psychiatric survivors, to share leadership and organizing skills, to strengthen community bonds, and to create coalitions with other marginalized groups (Finkler, 1997, 2009; Reaume, 2021). Psychiatric Survivor Pride Day was held almost annually for the remainder of the 1990s, with the events taking place in Parkdale, an area with numerous boarding homes and many psychiatric survivor residents (which has since been gentrified). Participants came together around issues of affordable and safe housing, as many boarding homes were crowded and unsafe (Finkler, 2009). Workshops were held to share information about tenants' rights, navigating social assistance benefits, policing, and forced psychiatric treatment (Finkler, 1997; Piepzna-Samarasinha, 2018). There were also clothing swaps, food, entertainment, and marches down Queen Street (Finkler, 1997; Piepzna-Samarasinha, 2018; Reaume, 2008). Such marches were an important way of creating community and raising the visibility of issues such as forced treatment, housing rights, and memorializing psychiatric survivors who had died. Regarding a march that went to a boarding home in

Parkdale where six psychiatric survivors were killed in a house fire, Piepzna-Samarasinha (2018) states:

> The impact of seeing a bunch of nuts being a people, marching with dignity and resistance to mourn our dead, assert our humanity, and demand our right to be Crazy without punishment, had a huge impact on both those marching and those watching.
>
> (pp. 86–87)

Piepzna-Samarasinha (2018) remembers the organizing of Psychiatric Survivor Pride Day events in the 1990s as predominantly led by queer, Indigenous, Black, and racialized women and as intersectional and coalitional:

> Like in much psych survivor organizing, there were white, cis, straight Crazy dudes who sometimes tried to dominate, in my memory the majority of the participants were Black, brown, and Native women, many of whom were queer. We were led by [Chava], who was great at telling a white Crazy dude to stop yelling at a brown Crazy woman. It was from her queer brown craziness that the idea of a Psychiatric Survivor Pride Day had come - queer people had come up with the idea of Pride, not shame, she said, and psych survivors often both were queer and had a lot of shame to overcome.
>
> (p. 86)

In the early 2000s, Psychiatric Survivor Pride Day underwent several name changes, eventually settling on Mad Pride in 2002 (Reaume, 2008), a name that Piepzna-Samarasinha (2018) attributes to Peggy-Gail Dehal-Ramson (p. 87). Since then, Mad Pride has taken place regularly but sporadically, in keeping with community interest and organizing capacity. At times it has been held annually, while at other times there has been a hiatus of several years in between events. Mad Pride in the 2000s has seen marches with the now iconic "bed push," in which participants don hospital gowns and restraints and push a hospital bed down the street to raise awareness about forced treatment and to "visibly commandeer and collectively re-occupy experiences typically controlled and defined by psychiatrists and other health care professionals" (Schrader et al., 2013, p. 62).[7] Starting in 2000, Mad Pride also included Geoffrey Reaume's wall tour of the patient-built brick wall at the Centre for Addiction and Mental Health, formerly the Provincial Lunatic Asylum. These walls, of which only a portion remain, were built by unpaid asylum patients in 1860. Reaume's tours highlighted the issue of unpaid patient labour and made the wall "relevant to people today who appreciate it as a memorial to people who have been previously forgotten and unmarked in public monuments" (Reaume, 2010, p. 134). Mad Pride continues to be significant in terms of community building, empowerment, and creating social change. Mad Pride has become international, with events taking place in many countries including France (Haigh, 2016), Ireland, Britain, and Ghana (Nabbali, 2013), Mexico, Chile, Korea, and the United States (Oaks, 2022).

BLACK POWER, MAD RESISTANCE

It is important to look beyond the Mad movement for some of the origins of Mad Studies. Mad movements were influenced by, and intersected with, other activist movements of the time. Further, Mad resistance was taking place in different ways outside of white, cis, heterosexual-dominated spaces. As Schalk (2022) explains, Black activists and cultural workers often address issues of madness and disability in ways that are grounded in understandings of white supremacy rather than focusing on pride, identity, and rights-based frameworks. There have been calls for a "more capacious recognition of the activist movements to which disability scholars should be accountable" (Minich, 2016, para 7) and the same can be said for Mad Studies scholars. Schalk's (2022) work on the Black Panther Party's resistance to psychiatric oppression is key in this regard.

The Black Panther Party (BPP) was founded in 1966 in Oakland, California, and can be seen as part of the wider Black Power movement of the 1960s and 1970s. The advent of Black Power on the heels of the civil rights movement can be seen as a turning away from a "politics of respectability" towards a "politics of rage," one that demonstrates a "mobilization of madness in black radical traditions of the 1960s" (Bruce, 2021, p. 24). At its height, BPP had chapters across the nation, as well as one in Algeria (Johnson, 1998). The BPP worked towards Black liberation, including issues of food security, housing, education, police violence, and reparations for slavery (Black Panther Party, 1966). Shalk (2022) shows how the BPP's ideology challenged psychiatrization in that "overmedicalization" of disability, whether physical, mental, or psychiatric, "depoliticized and individualized these experiences in ways that obscured the effect of the social and political on people's bodyminds, especially those from oppressed groups, who are more likely to be subject to state violence" (pp. 48–49).

Further, Schalk (2022) details collaborations between the BPP and various psychiatric survivor groups in the 1970s who were protesting psychiatric oppression in hospitals. The Party also published articles in their newspaper on forced drugging and institutionalization as well as labour issues such as unpaid work done by psychiatric patients (pp. 50–51). The BPP made connections between involuntary psychiatric commitment and prison incarceration, looking at how psychiatric drugs were used in prisons to control and manage inmate behaviour, particularly those who were activists (p. 53). They drew attention to how issues of psychiatric commitment and prison incarceration are racialized, in that these institutions operate together "to segregate, confine, and control Black people" (Schalk, 2022, p. 55). The BPP also challenged the practice of psychosurgery (brain surgery aimed at changing the recipient's behaviour), publishing articles about plans to perform it in prisons and in hospitals, targeting those who were seen as violent. The BPP drew attention to how this would disproportionately affect Black patients and inmates due to racist associations between violence and Blackness (Schalk, 2022). As Schalk's work demonstrates, there are many examples of resistance to psychiatric oppression in the work of the Black Panthers. It is therefore a necessary place to look for some of the origins of Mad Studies.

MAD RESISTANCE IN GAY LIBERATION AND TRANS ACTIVISM

Gay and trans activism of the 1960s and 1970s was multivocal and intersected with other leftist movements of the time (Ferguson, 2019). Gay and trans activists fought psychiatric oppression, and we can therefore look for some origins of Mad Studies in their struggles for social justice. The classification of homosexuality as a mental illness in the *Diagnostic and Statistical Manual of Mental Disorders* (DSM) is an obvious example of psychiatric oppression and is often held up as evidence that psychiatry is a form of social control that enforces social norms. Correspondingly, its declassification in 1973 is seen as a major accomplishment of the gay liberation movement. As I have explained in more detail elsewhere, one strand of gay activism employed a single-issue politic to fight for the declassification of homosexuality, ultimately serving to bolster psychiatry's legitimacy in some ways (Lewis, 2016; Pilling, 2022). However, there were other gay, lesbian, and trans activist voices and priorities at play that resisted psychiatry more broadly and were more in line with the coalitional politics of the times (Lewis, 2016; Pilling, 2022). There are many examples of Mad resistance that can be seen in these broader, coalitional forms of gay, lesbian, and trans activism in the 1960s and 1970s, and the following will highlight only a few.

While some American gay and lesbian activists were focused on declassification and used assimilationist strategies to reach their goals, others embraced notions of madness and insanity as liberational ways of knowing and being (Lewis, 2016). For such activists, "madness circulated not just as an object of analysis but also as a resource for critique and action; repudiating reason and sanity was often as integral to progressive sexual and gender politics as articulating solidarity with the insane" (Lewis, 2016, p. 87). Like the Black Panthers, some gay activists saw connections between prisons and psychiatric institutions, with some viewing them as "equivalent institutions" (Lewis, 2016, p. 106).

Trans activists were also active in Mad resistance. Stonewall activists in 1969 who fought back against police violence were led by trans women of colour. Accounts of Stonewall and other activism taking place at this time have been whitewashed, which

> elides the ways in which queer politics were emerging as ways to engage anti-poverty and anti-racism. For gay rights to advance an argument of singularity and the uniformity of queer struggles, it had to disappear trans and queer of color activism as linchpins between a variety of political struggles.
>
> (Ferguson, 2019, p. 44)

Gay rights' 'argument of singularity' also had to disappear disability and madness. Disability and madness were central in the lives of Stonewall activists such as trans feminine people of colour Marsha P. Johnson and Sylvia Rivera and the erasure of such is consistent with the ways in which queer disabled and Mad people are "written out of history in a way that is a constant, violent, intentional forgetting, by both those who explicitly want us dead and nondisabled Left and queer movements" (Piepzna-Samarasinha, 2019, p. 57). Piepzna-Samarasinha (2019) notes that Johnson and Rivera both struggled with suicidality, trauma, and distress and were commonly seen as "crazy" (p.59). In the early 1970s, Rivera and Johnson founded Street Transvestite Action Revolutionaries (STAR), a coalition of activists focused on providing housing and food, particularly to gay and trans youth (Feinberg, 2006). In Rivera's words, "STAR was for the street gay people, the street homeless people, and anybody that needed help at that time" (Rivera quoted in Feinberg, 2006). Rivera and Johnson, who both had experiences of homelessness and sex work, created shelters (a trailer truck and eventually a building called Star House) for those who needed a place to live (Feinberg, 2006). Piepzna-Samarasinha (2019) suggests that Rivera and Johnson's actions can be viewed as an example of the "crip kindness" that can sometimes be found in disabled and Mad communities:

> What would it mean to examine neurodiversity/suicidality, sadness, and complex post-traumatic stress disorder (CPTSD) in Johnson and other Stonewall warriors' lives as not just tragic disability and struggle, but also as the source of some of their gifts? When I look, as a Mad nonbinary femme of color, at Marsha and Sylvia's refusal of respectability politics, their radical kindness and openness to anyone coming through STAR House – including multiply marginalized street queens and trans women and other trans people, poor and of color, who no doubt were seen as "crazy," "too much," and shunned from other queer communities – I see a kind of "crip kindness" I have often witnessed, especially in radical mental health circles, where we are firm in our refusal to throw people away because of our own experiences of madness and being shunned.
>
> (p. 59)

STAR's activism can be seen as peer support or mutual aid, which has deep roots in communities who cannot rely on the state such as sex workers, queer and trans people, and racialized and Indigenous communities. STAR's work also shows intersecting priorities with psychiatric survivor movements, in terms of anti-poverty activism and employing an ethos of peer support. As this section has shown, there are many intersections and overlaps between gay, lesbian, and trans activism and psychiatric survivor movements.

THE EMERGENCE OF MAD STUDIES WITHIN ACADEMIA

Mad Studies disrupts many taken for granted assumptions about experiences of madness and distress and how to respond to them. As will be discussed in more detail in Chapter 2, many things that are now accepted as common sense about madness are rooted in colonial, Eurocentric ways of knowing that date back to the formation of the psy disciplines. Mad Studies challenges and interrupts foundational ideologies of the psy disciplines, which encompasses Psychiatry and Psychology as well as allied health disciplines such as Nursing, Social Work, and beyond. As such, the establishment of Mad Studies as an academic field is contested from all sides. Those who are invested in the psy disciplines resist madness as an analytic that challenges the authority of the psy disciplines and the expertise of psy professionals. Like other marginalized fields such as feminist, critical race, disability, and queer studies, Mad studies and Mad scholars can be subject to ridicule and attack from those who resent Mad agency and critiques of dominant ways of thinking (Costa & Ross, 2022). On the other hand, some Mad activists have legitimate concerns that academicizing Mad knowledge will result in its co-option and departure from community priorities (Archibald, 2024; Ingram, 2016). Despite its contested status, Mad Studies has established itself within academia and has grown exponentially since the turn of the century.

Before Mad Studies was named as such, there were courses being taught about Mad people's history beginning in the early 2000s (Reaume, 2006, 2019; Reville, 2013). Since then, the number of Mad Studies courses has increased in number and broadened in content and scope (Lefrançois & Peddle, 2022). At the same time, a growing number of scholars and writers were creating works about madness, building on the ideas, concepts, and practices circulating in Mad movements.[8] This led to the use of "Mad Studies" and "Madness Studies" as names to describe this emergent body of work. The publishing of *Mad Matters: A Critical Reader in Canadian Mad Studies* in 2013 was a defining moment in the establishment of Mad Studies and solidified the use of "Mad Studies" over "Madness Studies" (though both are still in use). There are other texts that have served to entrench Mad Studies as an academic field of study, including the more recent *Routledge International Handbook of Mad Studies*, published in 2022. Mad Studies has always been an interdisciplinary and multidisciplinary field of study. Given the lack of post-secondary Mad Studies programs, most Mad Studies scholars are necessarily trained in other fields and bring these perspectives to bear on their work. The following sections highlight two areas of study in which Mad Studies origins can be found, however, there are many more.

MAD STUDIES ORIGINS IN DISABILITY STUDIES

Mad Studies has roots in Disability Studies and has sometimes been positioned as *being of* Disability Studies, though it is now seen as a field in its own right. Much debate surrounds the interconnections between Disability Studies and Mad Studies, what they are, and what they should be (Beresford, 2000; Beresford & Russo, 2016; Church, 2015; Jones & Brown, 2013; Morgan, 2022; Nabbali, 2009; Stefan, 2018; Thorneycroft, 2020). Whether madness should be considered a disability is also contentious (Spandler et al., 2015). That said, Mad Studies often finds a home within Disability Studies in the academy. Some Mad Studies scholars are located institutionally within Disability Studies programs and many Mad Studies courses are taught within Disability Studies. Toronto Metropolitan University's School of Disability Studies is noteworthy in the development of Mad Studies and Mad pedagogy, with Mad Studies courses being taught there since the early 2000s (Church, 2013, 2015; Landry & Church, 2016; Snyder et al., 2019; Reaume, 2006, 2019; Reville, 2013).

Likewise, Disability Studies and Mad Studies share some intellectual traditions and frameworks. Most notably, the positioning of disability as social and political (rather than as strictly medical) has been influential in Mad Studies (Beresford, 2002; Lefrançois & Peddle, 2022). Disability Studies exposes the ways in which social environments create disability rather than locating disability in 'disordered' bodies (for example, a wheelchair user is disabled by a lack of ramps and elevators). A key sticking point for Mad Studies has been Disability Studies' separation of 'impairment' as an embodied state from 'disability' as a social and political phenomenon produced by the built environment and ableist social attitudes and practices. Mad Studies scholars have critiqued the notion of impairment for reifying the medicalization of distress and reinforcing biological essentialism (Beresford & Wallcraft, 1997; Nabbali, 2009). Mad Studies has been influenced by Disability Studies' analyses of normalcy and how disabled people become pathologized as deviant and abnormal (Lefrançois & Peddle, 2022). Disability Studies' critiques of medicalized notions of disabled bodies as deficient, biologically inferior, and in need of cure, correction, or elimination has likewise been significant (Clare, 2017). Disability Studies exposes and challenges ableist beliefs about disabled people as tragic, pitiable, burdensome, or as brave and inspirational 'supercrips' (Young, 2014; Wood, 2012) and such critiques have aided in the formulation of the concept of sanism in Mad Studies (Lefrançois & Peddle, 2022). Disability Studies counters the widespread idea that disabled lives are not worth living and instead sees disability as a necessary form of human biodiversity (Garland-Thomson, 2015; McBryde Johnson, 2003), an idea that is reflected in conceptualizations of Mad pride.

There are limitations to Disability Studies' capacity to address madness. Indeed, the focus of Disability Studies has been on physical disability, to the exclusion of madness and chronic illness. Further, Disability Studies tends to overlook the types of conditions that most affect poor and racialized communities, such as chronic conditions caused by environmental racism (Kafer, 2013; Schalk, 2022). Some white Disability Studies scholars have argued that ableism is the last bastion of socially acceptable forms of discrimination, showing a lack of understanding of how ableism is mutually constitutive with other forms of oppression like racism, as well as the ongoing severity and social acceptance of such. This lack of intersectional analysis has limited Disability Studies' relevance to the lives of disabled Indigenous, Black, and racialized people (Jarman, 2011; Mollow, 2006). Bell's (2006) intervention into the field argues that like other areas of study, Disability Studies centres whiteness as the unexamined norm. He explains that this is not an exclusion of people of colour, rather, people of colour are treated "as if they were white people; as if there are no critical exigencies involved in being people of color that might necessitate these individuals understanding and negotiating disability in a different way from their white counterparts" (p. 272). As Pickens (2019) points out, Disability Studies "borrows heavily from the gains of critical race studies and women's studies" and, therefore, "race is always already embedded in scholastic discussions of disability" (p. 7). And yet, as she goes on to state,

> The principles of critical race studies tend to have a penumbral presence because disability studies rarely engages whiteness as a social position and often thinks of Blackness as a contribution rather than part of its construction …. As long as whiteness remains the normative racial category, investigations of disability that do not address whiteness directly leave open crucial lacunae.
>
> (p. 7)

These limitations of Disability Studies have informed Mad Studies and are part of its origins. Some Mad scholarship has perpetuated some of these issues, including the privileging of white scholars and activists' contributions, and the centring of whiteness as the unmarked and unexamined norm. A recent trend of adding the word "critical" to Mad Studies aims to rectify these issues and draw a distinction between Mad Studies scholarship that embraces a white-centric single-issue politic and that which employs intersectional, critical race, and decolonial perspectives. Lefrançois and Peddle (2022) resist this trend, arguing that it "erase[s] the contributions of MPOC [Mad people of colour] from the inception of mad studies, as well as … the important critical race and postcolonial theorizing that has been integral to mad studies from its beginning" (p. 467). They suggest an alternate strategy of "continu[ing] to use and develop mad theory and a mad studies that both makes visible and refuses these erasures" (p. 467). Whether or not the prefix 'critical' takes hold, it is crucial that Mad Studies continues to do just that.

Arising from 1960s feminist movements, Gender and Women's Studies is an interdisciplinary field that tends to house all manner of critical scholars, especially those working in Sexuality Studies, queer theory, Trans Studies, critical race studies, postcolonial, and transnational feminisms, and to a lesser extent, Disability Studies. Since the establishment of academic Women's Studies programs in the 1970s, there have been continuous tensions regarding who and what should be included in the field, especially when it comes to trans inclusion, critical race studies, and disability (Beauchamp & D'Harlingue, 2012; Bhavnani, 1997; Brown, 1997; Garland-Thomson, 2005). In the early 2000s, many programs began to change their names from 'Women's Studies' to various configurations that include the word 'gender' and other terms such as 'feminism,' 'sexuality,' 'race,' and 'social justice.' These name changes reflect shifts in the field that challenge bioessentialist definitions of womanhood and widen the focus on women's experiences to include analyses of gender as an analytic (rather than as an identity category). These name changes also make explicit the field's intersectional understandings of sexism and misogyny as mutually constitutive with other forms of oppression.

Some of Mad Studies' roots can be seen within women of colour feminisms, postcolonial, and decolonial feminist theories (Johnk, 2021; Lefrançois & Peddle, 2022). These have influenced Mad Studies' analyses of psychiatry as a tool of colonization, the disproportionate number of racialized and Indigenous people in psychiatric institutions, and racism within psychiatric survivor activism (Lefrançois & Peddle, 2022). Ideas found within women of colour feminisms such as challenges to the mind/body Cartesian dualism can be seen as precursors to Mad Studies disruptions to this binary (Johnk, 2021). Likewise, Black feminist thought on intersectionality

(Collins, 1990; Combahee River Collective, 1977; Crenshaw, 1989) has influenced Mad Studies understandings of sanism as mutually constitutive with racism and other forms of oppression (Abdillahi et al., 2017; Meerai et al., 2016; Pilling, 2021).

Mad Studies' roots can also be seen in feminist analyses of patriarchal oppression in psychiatry dating back to the 1970s onwards. Some feminists argue that psychiatry is a form of social control that pathologizes women and blames them for the impacts of sexism and misogyny (Busfield, 1996; Ehrenreich & English, 1978; Showalter, 1985; Smith & David, 1975; Ussher, 1992). Feminists also analyze gendered psychiatric constructs such as hysteria, which positioned white, middle to upper class Victorian women as inherently ill due to their reproductive systems (Ehrenreich & English, 1978; Smith-Rosenberg, 1985). This feminist work influenced Mad Studies' understanding of psychiatry as a gendered form of social control. Contemporary Mad theorizing includes analyses of gendered diagnoses such as the feminization of depression (Ussher, 2011), premenstrual dysphoric disorder, and female sexual interest/arousal disorder (Cohen & Hartmaan, 2023). Other contemporary Mad feminist critiques of normative femininity include analyses of the role of psychiatry in enforcing gender norms (Cohen & Hartmann, 2023; Rimke, 2018). As will be discussed further in Chapter 3, feminist critiques of positivism and hierarchies of types of evidence can be seen as influential in psychiatric survivor research. Feminist methodological interventions that established the value of women's lived experience as an authoritative source of knowledge can be seen in Mad Studies' valuing of Mad knowledge and efforts to achieve epistemic justice for Mad people, a concept that is discussed further in Chapter 2 (Morrow, 2017). Feminist, queer, and critical race scholars who theorize gender, sexuality, and race as social constructs with material consequences (Butler, 1990; Omi & Winant, 1993) can be seen as instrumental in Mad Studies' understandings of madness as rooted in social processes.

Tools of the feminist movement can also be seen as influencing Mad praxis. For example, feminists engaged in consciousness-raising groups, which provided mutual support while raising awareness that individual problems are rooted in structural inequities, or, as the feminist catch phrase goes, 'the personal is political.' These groups can be seen as influencing the Mad practice of peer support, which provides non-professionalized support by and for people who have experienced distress and mental health systems (Guzmán Martínez et al., 2021). However, feminist activism and scholarship has had a fraught relationship to Mad activism and scholarship. Feminist efforts to establish women's mental health services have moved away from earlier feminist critiques of psychiatry and have largely ignored Mad analyses of the oppressive nature of such services (Morrow, 2017). Some feminist theories have been seen as elitist, academic, and grounded in the writing of feminist mental health professionals rather than in the lives of people who have experienced mental health systems (Guzmán Martínez et al., 2021; Morrow, 2017). However, given its interdisciplinary and critical nature, Gender and Women's Studies programs remain an important location within academia where scholars can engage with Mad Studies and create Mad knowledge.

Mad Studies has been firmly established as a field of academic study, and yet, it is precariously situated within academia, as evidenced by the recent dismantling of the world's first Master's program in Mad Studies after only three years (Macintosh, 2023). The post-secondary sector's adoption of a neoliberal business model has resulted in cuts to programs and marginalized areas of study are always most at risk. Many programs face demands to downsize the number of courses on offer and cut program requirements, curtailing opportunities to develop cutting-edge courses in newer fields such as Mad Studies. Universities increasingly rely on precarious contract labour, cutting the number of secure tenure-track positions. This inhibits the growth and sustainability of Mad Studies by reducing the possibility of secure jobs for Mad Studies scholars and thereby the capacity to offer Mad Studies courses as an ongoing component of degree programs.[9] Mad Studies' place in academia is far from secure, and yet great progress has been made since its (more formal) inception as a field of study at the turn of the century. As it becomes more entrenched within academia, efforts to dilute, co-opt, and politically neutralize it will no doubt increase. However, it is important for Mad Studies to remain generative rather than dogmatic in its attempt to remain radical. This will be a difficult balance to strike.

This chapter provided a brief outline of some of the origins of Mad Studies as well as its emergence in academia. This chapter also explored the importance of resisting the whitewashing and cis-heterosexualizing of Mad Studies and its origins. I hope that accounts of the origins of Mad Studies proliferate in years to come, including Indigenous accounts of how Mad resistance may be in conversation with Indigenous ways of knowing, historical works that unearth queer and trans liberation's intersections with resistance to psychiatric oppression, Mad readings of works by queer and trans Indigenous, Black, and racialized people, archival work that details the contributions of queer, trans, Indigenous, Black, and racialized Mad activists to the Mad movement, and additional works that read against the grain of institutional records for the stories of queer and trans people.

Recommended resources

Jackson, V. (2002). In our own voice: African-American stories of oppression, survival and recovery in mental health systems. *International Journal of Narrative Therapy and Community Work, 2*, 11–31.

Lewis, A. J. (2016). "We are certain of our own insanity": Antipsychiatry and the gay liberation movement, 1968–1980. *Journal of the History of Sexuality, 25*(1), 83–113. https://doi.org/10.7560/jhs25104

Madness Canada Archives: https://madnesscanada.com/resources/archives/

MPA Documentary Collective. (2013). The Inmates Are Running the Asylum [Film]. Madness Canada. https://madnesscanada.com/mad-cities/the-inmates-are-running-the-asylum/

NOTES

1 My focus in this chapter is on Canada and the United States. However, it is important to note that there was a significant and influential movement of the same era in the United Kingdom, and it remains a major hub for Mad activism and scholarship today (Blayney, 2022; Campbell, 2005, 2022; Gallagher, 2017, 2021; Sapouna & O'Donnell, 2017; Spandler, 2006, 2020; Spandler & Carr, 2021). Likewise, there are movements across the world including (but not limited to) Latin America (Burstow & Castillo, 2019; Madrid, 2023; Quiroz, 2022), Africa (Eromosele, 2022; Nabbali, 2013), Japan (Kirihara, 2022), and New Zealand (O'Hagan & Beresford, 2022).

2 By "whitewashing" and "cis-heterosexualizing," I mean centring white, cisgender (i.e. non-trans), heterosexual histories, concerns, values, and contributions and using whiteness, cisgenderism, and heterosexuality as unmarked norms.

3 The abolition vs. reform is a false binary. Abolitionists recognize that it is a long-term project that requires big shifts in the organization of society and some work on goals that may be characterized as reformist as a means of making more immediate change to the system that make it more liveable and less violent. For a more nuanced discussion of abolition and reform see Ben-Moshe, 2020.

4 Likewise, Mad Studies should not be conflated with anti-psychiatry or critical psychiatry. Mad Studies is broad enough to include these perspectives but is not defined or eclipsed by them. For a more nuanced discussion of the differences between Mad Studies, anti-psychiatry, and critical psychiatry see Reaume, 2022.

5 *Madness Network News* still exists today in an online format: https://madness-networknews.com

6 To be clear, ideas such as safe, affordable housing for all and peer support are not radical, but they are positioned as such in relation to the status quo, especially in contemporary times.

7 Nabbali (2013) attributes the first bed push to Mad Pride activists in Britain in 2005, who pushed "a hospital bed from Millview Psychiatric Hospital in Brighton to the original site of 'Bedlam,' the longest-running psychiatric institution while being chased by a giant syringe" (p. 185).

8 Lefrançois & Peddle (2022) attribute the conceptualization of Mad Studies to Lucy Costa, Erick Fabris, Rachel Gorman, Richard Ingram, Geoffrey Reaume, and Jijian Voronka. This list is not meant to be exhaustive and only includes Canadian scholars based in Toronto, Ontario.

9 For example, during my three-year limited term (i.e. non-permanent) appointment at the University of Windsor I developed and taught a Mad Studies course called Disability, Madness and Social Justice which, to my knowledge, was the first and only Mad Studies course to be taught there. After two years of offering it as a special topics course, I attained formal inclusion of the course in the undergraduate course calendar and by its third offering the course reached enrollment capacity. However, the course became defunct upon my departure.

REFERENCES

Abdillahi, I., Meerai, S., & Poole, J. (2017). When the suffering is compounded: Towards anti-Black sanism. In S. Wehbi &

H. Parada (Eds.), *Reimagining anti-oppression social work practice* (pp. 109–122). Canadian Scholars Press.

Adame, A. L., Morsey, M., Bassman, R., Yates, K. (2017). *Exploring identities of psychiatric survivor therapists: Beyond us and them.* Palgrave Macmillan. https://doi.org/10.1057/978-1-137-58492-2_2

Archibald, L. (2024). Maintaining the fidelity of Mad Studies (An ode to Mad Studies 2). *Asylum*, 31(1), 16–17.

Beauchamp, T., & D'Harlingue, B. (2012). Beyond additions and exceptions: The category of transgender and new pedagogical approaches for women's studies. *Feminist Formations*, 24(2), 25–51. https://doi.org/10.1353/ff.2012.0020

Beckman, L. & Davies, M. (2013). Democracy is a very radical idea. In B. A. LeFrançois, R. Menzies, & G. Reaume, *Mad matters: A critical reader in Canadian Mad Studies* (pp. 49–63). Canadian Scholars Press.

Bell, C. (2006). Introducing white disability studies. In L. J. Davis (Ed.), *The Disability Studies reader* (2nd ed., pp. 275–282). Routledge.

Ben-Moshe, L. (2020). *Decarcerating disability: Deinstitutionalization and prison abolition.* University of Minnesota Press. https://doi.org/10.5749/j.ctv10vm2vw

Beresford, P. & Russo, J. (2016). Supporting the sustainability of Mad Studies and preventing its co-option. *Disability & Society*, 31(2), 270–274. https://doi.org/10.1080/09687599.2016.1145380

Beresford, P. (2000). What have madness and psychiatric system survivors got to do with disability and disability studies? *Disability & Society*, 15(1), 167–172. https://doi.org/10.1080/09687590025838

Beresford, P. (2002). Thinking about "mental health": Towards a social model. *Journal of Mental Health*, 11(6), 581–584. https://doi.org/10.1080/09638230020023921

Bhavnani, K. K. (1997). Women's studies and its interconnection with "race", ethnicity and sexuality. In V. Robinson & D. Richardson (Eds.), *Introducing women's studies: Feminist theory and practice* (pp. 27–53). New York University Press. https://doi.org/10.1007/978-1-349-25726-3_2

Blayney, S. (2022). Activist sources and the survivor movement. In C. Millard and J. Wallis (Eds.), *Sources in the history of psychiatry, from 1800 to the present*. Routledge. https://doi.org/10.4324/9781003087694-11

Brown, W. (1997). The impossibility of women's studies. *Differences: A Journal of Feminist Cultural Studies, 9*(3), 79–101. https://doi.org/10.1215/10407391-9-3-79

Black Panther Party. (1966). *The Black Panther Party Ten-Point Program*. BlackPast. www.blackpast.org/african-american-history/primary-documents-african-american-history/black-panther-party-ten-point-program-1966/

Bruce, L. M. J. (2021). *How to go mad without losing your mind: Madness and black radical creativity*. Duke University Press. https://doi.org/10.2307/j.ctv1ks0hp4

Burstow, B. & Castillo, T. (2019). "Activism is my real job": The Mad movement in Chile dialogue with Tatiana Castillo. In B. Burstow (Ed.), *The revolt against psychiatry: A counterhegemonic dialogue* (pp. 109–119). Springer. https://doi.org/10.1007/978-3-030-23331-0_8

Burstow, B. & Weitz, D. (1988). *Shrink resistant: The struggle against psychiatry in Canada*. New Star Books.

Busfield, J. (1996). *Men, women, and madness: Understanding gender and mental disorder*. New York University Press.

Butler, J. (1990). *Gender trouble: Feminism and the subversion of identity*. Routledge.

Campbell, P. (2005). From little acorns: The mental health service user movement. In A. Bell and P. Lindley (Eds.), *Beyond the water towers: The unfinished revolution in mental health services 1985–2005* (pp. 73–82). The Sainsbury Centre for Mental Health.

Campbell, P. (2022). Speaking for ourselves: An early UK survivor activist's account. In P. Beresford and J. Russo (Eds.), *The Routledge international handbook of Mad Studies* (pp. 57–59). Routledge. https://doi.org/10.4324/9780429465444-8

Chamberlin, J. (1978). *On our own: Patient controlled alternatives to the mental health system*. McGraw-Hill.

Church, K. (2013). Making madness matter in academic practice. In B. A. LeFrançois, R. Menzies, & G. Reaume,

Mad matters: A critical reader in Canadian Mad Studies (pp. 181–190). Canadian Scholars Press.

Church, K. (2015). 'It's complicated': Blending disability and Mad Studies in the corporatising university. In H. Spandler, J. Anderson, & B. Sapey (Eds.), *Madness, distress and the politics of disablement* (pp. 261–270). Policy Press. https://doi.org/10.46692/9781447314592.020

Clare, E. (2017). *Brilliant imperfection: Grappling with cure.* Duke University Press. https://doi.org/10.1515/9780822373520

Cohen, B. M. & Hartmann, R. (2023). The "feminisation" of psychiatric discourse: A Marxist analysis of women's roles in neoliberal society. *Journal of Sociology, 59*(2), 349–364. https://doi.org/10.1177/14407833211043570

Collins, P. H. (1990). *Black feminist thought: Knowledge, consciousness, and the politics of empowerment.* Routledge.

Combahee River Collective. (1977). *Combahee River collective statement.* BlackPast. www.blackpast.org/african-american-history/combahee-river-collective-statement-1977/

Costa, L. & Ross, L. (2023). Mad Studies genealogy and praxis. *International Mad Studies Journal, 1*(1), e1–8. https://doi.org/10.58544/imsj.v1i1.5239

Crenshaw, K. (1989). Demarginalizing the intersection of race and sex: A Black feminist critique of antidiscrimination doctrine, feminist theory and antiracist politics. *University of Chicago Legal Forum,* 1989(1), 139–167.

Daley, A. (2021). Narrating genders in psychiatric inpatient chart documentation. In A. Daley & M. D. Pilling (Eds.), *Interrogating psychiatric narratives of madness: Documented lives* (pp. 57–86). Palgrave Macmillan. https://doi.org/10.1007/978-3-030-83692-4_3

Deerinwater, J., Ho, S., Thompson, V., Wong, A., Erevelles, N., & Morrow, M. (2023). A conversation on disability justice and intersectionality. In *Handbook of disability: Critical thought and social change in a globalizing world* (pp. 1–22). Springer Nature. https://doi.org/10.1007/978-981-16-1278-7_95-1

Ehrenreich, B. & English, D. (1978). *For her own good: 150 years of the experts' advice to women.* Anchor Press.

Eromosele, F. (2022). Madness, decolonization and mental health activism in Africa. In P. Beresford and J. Russo (Eds.), *The Routledge international handbook of Mad Studies* (pp. 327–339). Routledge. https://doi.org/10.4324/9780429465444-38

Feinberg, L. (2006, September 24). *Street transvestite action revolutionaries.* Workers World. www.workers.org/2006/us/lavender-red-73/

Fernando, S. (2010). *Mental health, race and culture.* Palgrave Macmillan. https://doi.org/10.1007/978-1-137-01368-2

Finkler, L. (1997). Psychiatric survivor pride day: Community organizing with psychiatric survivors. *Osgoode Hall Law Journal, 35*(3/4), 763–772. https://doi.org/10.60082/2817-5069.1596

Finkler, L. (2009, July 15). Mad Pride: A movement for social change. *The Consumer/Survivor Information Resource Centre of Toronto Bulletin, 398*, 2–3.

Ferguson, R. A. (2019). *One-Dimensional Queer.* Polity Press.

Gallagher, M. (2017). From asylum to action in Scotland: the emergence of the Scottish Union of Mental Patients, 1971–2. *History of Psychiatry, 28*(1), 101–114. https://doi.org/10.1177/0957154X16678124

Gallagher, M. (2021). Making public their use of history: Reflections on the history of collective action by psychiatric patients, the Oor Mad History Project and Survivors History Group. In R. Ellis, S. Kendal, & S. Taylor (Eds.), *Voices in the history of madness: Personal and professional perspectives on mental health and illness* (pp. 359–381). Springer. https://doi.org/10.1007/978-3-030-69559-0_17

Garland-Thomson, R. (2005). Feminist disability studies. *Signs: Journal of women in Culture and Society, 30*(2), 1557–1587. https://doi.org/10.1086/423352

Garland-Thomson, R. (2015). Human biodiversity conservation: A consensual ethical principle. *The American Journal of Bioethics, 15*(6), 13–15. https://doi.org/10.1080/15265161.2015.1028663

Guzmán Martínez, G., Pujal i Llombart, M., Mora Malo, E., & García Dauder, D. (2021). Antecedentes feministas de los grupos de apoyo mutuo en el movimiento loco: Un análisis histórico-crítico. *Salud Colectiva*, *17*, e3274. https://doi.org/10.18294/sc.2021.3274

Haigh, S. (2016). "Mad Pride France": Disability, mental distress, and citizenship. *Journal of Literary & Cultural Disability Studies*, *10*(2), 191–206. https://doi.org/10.3828/jlcds.2016.16

Hectors, A. (2023). Homosexuality in the DSM: A critique of depathologisation and heteronormativity. *New Zealand Sociology*, *38*(1), 18–28.

Howell, A. & Voronka, J. (2012). Introduction: The politics of resilience and recovery in mental health care. *Studies in Social Justice*, *6*(1), 1–7. https://doi.org/10.26522/ssj.v6i1.1065

Hylton, A. (2024). *Madness: Race and insanity in a Jim Crow asylum*. Grand Central Publishing.

Ingram, R. A. (2016). Doing mad studies: Making (non) sense together. *Intersectionalities: A Global Journal of Social Work Analysis, Research, Polity, and Practice*, *5*(3), 11–17.

Jackson, V. (2002). In our own voice: African-American stories of oppression, survival and recovery in mental health systems. *International Journal of Narrative Therapy and Community Work*, *2*, 11–31.

Jarman, M. (2011). Coming up from underground: Uneasy dialogues at the intersections of race, mental illness, and disability studies. In C. Bell (Ed.), *Blackness and disability: Critical examinations and cultural interventions* (pp. 9–29). Michigan State University Press.

Johnk, L. (2021). *Shifting roots: Reimagining the genealogical roots of Disability Studies and Mad Studies through women of color feminisms* [Doctoral dissertation, Oregon State University]. ScholarsArchive@OSU.

Johnson, O. (1998). Explaining the demise of the Black Panther Party. In C. E. Jones (Ed.), *The Black Panther Party (reconsidered)* (pp. 391–409). Black Classic Press.

Jones, N. & Brown, R. (2013). The absence of psychiatric C/S/X perspectives in academic discourse: Consequences and implications. *Disability Studies Quarterly*, *33*(1). https://doi.org/10.18061/dsq.v33i1.3433

Joseph, A. J. (2014). A prescription for violence: The legacy of colonization in contemporary forensic mental health and the production of difference. *Critical Criminology, 22,* 273–292. https://doi.org/10.1007/s10612-013-9208-1

Joseph, A. J. (2019). Contemporary forms of legislative imprisonment and colonial violence in forensic mental health. In A. Daley, L. Costa, & P. Beresford (Eds.), *Madness, violence, and power: A critical collection* (pp. 169–183). University of Toronto Press. https://doi.org/10.3138/9781442629981-017

Joseph, A. (2022). The subjects of oblivion: Subalterity, sanism, and racial erasure. In P. Beresford and J. Russo (Eds.), *The Routledge international handbook of Mad Studies* (pp. 135–141). Routledge. https://doi.org/10.4324/9780429465444-19

Kafer, A. (2013). *Feminist, queer, crip.* Indiana University Press.

Kalathil, J. (2013). "Hard to reach"? Racialized groups and mental health service user involvement. In P. Staddon (Ed.), *Mental health service users in research: Critical sociological perspectives* (pp. 121–133). Policy Press. https://doi.org/10.1332/policypress/9781447307334.003.0009

Kirihara, N. (2022). The social movement of people with psychosocial disabilities in Japan: Strategies for taking the struggle to academia. In P. Beresford and J. Russo (Eds.), *The Routledge international handbook of Mad Studies* (pp. 66–75). Routledge. https://doi.org/10.4324/9780429465444-11

Landry, D. (2023). Mad student organizing and the growth of Mad Studies in Canada. *Research Papers in Education, 38*(5), 763–782. https://doi.org/10.1080/02671522.2023.2219677

Landry, D. & Church, K. (2016). Teaching (like) crazy in a mad positive school: Exploring the charms of recursion. In J. Russo & A. Sweeney (Eds.), *Searching for a rose garden: Challenging psychiatry, fostering Mad Studies* (pp. 172–182). PCCS Books.

Lavallée, L. (2021, January 12). *Spirit injuries: Indigenous perspectives of mental health* [Video]. Network Environments for Indigenous Health Research Ontario Webinar,

Waakebiness-Bryce Institute for Indigenous Health, Dalla Lana School of Public Health, University of Toronto. YouTube. https://youtu.be/Jul3glN3UH4?si=tCyPM_y0wueRLJd0

LeFrançois, B. A. & Peddle, C. R. (2022). Mad studies, mad theory. In S. S. Shaikh, B. A. LeFrançois, & T. Macías (Eds.), *Critical social work praxis* (pp. 463–476). Fernwood Publishing.

Lewis, B. (2006). A mad fight: Psychiatry and disability activism. In L. J. Davis (Ed.), *The disability studies reader* (2nd ed., pp. 488–504). Routledge. https://doi.org/10.4324/9781315680668-14

Lewis, A. J. (2016). "We are certain of our own insanity": Antipsychiatry and the gay liberation movement, 1968–1980. *Journal of the History of Sexuality*, 25(1), 83–113. https://doi.org/10.7560/jhs25104

Macintosh, J. (2023). Ode to the MSc in Mad Studies. *Asylum*, 30(4), 6–7.

Madrid, J. C. C. (2023). Latin-American Mad Studies: Conceptual frameworks and research agenda. *Physis: Revista de Saúde Coletiva*, 32. https://doi.org/10.1590/S0103-73312022320403-en

McBryde Johnson, H. (2003). Unspeakable conversations. In C. M. Koggell (Ed.), *Moral issues in global perspective* (2nd Ed., Vol. 3, pp. 86–97). Broadview Press.

Meerai, S., Abdillahi, I., & Poole, J. (2016). An introduction to anti-Black sanism. *Intersectionalities: A Global Journal of Social Work Analysis, Research, Polity, and Practice*, 5(3), 18–35. https://doi.org/10.32920/21751496

Menzies, R., LeFrancois, B. A., & Reaume, G. (2013). Introducing Mad Studies. In B. A. LeFrançois, R. Menzies, & G. Reaume, *Mad matters: A critical reader in Canadian Mad Studies* (pp. 1–26). Canadian Scholars Press.

Minich, J. A. (2016) Enabling whom? Critical Disability Studies now. *Lateral*, 5(1). https://doi.org/10.25158/L5.1.9

Madness Canada. (n.d.). *Archives*. https://madnesscanada.com/resources/archives/

Mollow, A. (2006). "When Black women start going on Prozac": Race, gender, and mental illness in Meri Nana-Ama

Danquah's Willow weep for me. *Melus, 31*(3), 67–99. https://doi.org/10.1093/melus/31.3.67

Morrison, L. J. (2005). *Talking back to psychiatry: The psychiatric consumer/survivor/ex-patient movement.* Routledge. https://doi.org/10.4324/9780203958704

Morrow, M. (2017). Women and madness revisited: The promise of intersectional and Mad Studies frameworks. In M. Morrow & L. Malcoe (Eds.), *Critical inquiries for social justice in mental health* (pp. 33–59). University of Toronto Press. https://doi.org/10.3138/9781442619708-003

Morgan, H. (2022). Mad studies and disability studies. In P. Beresford and J. Russo (Eds.), *The Routledge international handbook of Mad Studies* (pp. 108–118). Routledge. https://doi.org/10.4324/9780429465444-16

MPA Documentary Collective. (2013). *The inmates are running the asylum* [Film]. Madness Canada. https://madnesscanada.com/mad-cities/the-inmates-are-running-the-asylum/

Nabbali, E. M. (2009). A "mad" critique of the social model of disability. *International Journal of Diversity in Organizations, Communities, and Nations, 9*(4), 1. https://doi.org/10.18848/1447-9532/cgp/v09i04/39702

Nabbali, E. M. (2013). "Mad" activism and its (Ghanaian?) future: A prolegomena to debate. *Trans-Scripts, 3,* 178–201.

Oaks, D. (2022, July 14). *July is both Disability Pride month and Mad Pride month: Happy Bastille Day!* Mad in America. www.madinamerica.com/2022/07/july-disability-mad-pride/

O'Hagan, M., & Beresford, P. (2022). Reflections on power, knowledge and change. In P. Beresford and J. Russo (Eds.), *The Routledge international handbook of Mad Studies* (pp. 30–33). Routledge. https://doi.org/10.4324/9780429465444-4

Omi, M. & Winant, H. (1993). On the theoretical concept of race. In C. McCarthy & W. Crichlow, G. Dimitriadis, & N. Dolby (Eds.), *Race identity and representation in education* (pp. 3–10). Routledge.

Pickens, T. A. (2019). *Black madness: Mad Blackness.* Duke University Press. https://doi.org/10.1515/9781478005506

Piepzna-Samarasinha, L. L. (2019). Disability justice/Stonewall's legacy, or: Love mad trans Black women when they are alive and dead, let their revolutions teach your resistance all the time. *QED: A Journal in GLBTQ Worldmaking*, 6(2), 54–62. https://doi.org/10.14321/qed.6.2.0054

Piepzna-Samarasinha, L. L. (2018). *Care Work: Dreaming Disability Justice*. Arsenal Pulp Press.

Pilling, M. D. (2021). Sexual violence and psychosis: Intersections of rape culture, sanism, and anti-Black sanism in psychiatric inpatient chart documentation. In A. Daley & M. D. Pilling (Eds.), *Interrogating psychiatric narratives of madness: Documented lives* (pp. 137–164). Palgrave Macmillan. https://doi.org/10.1080/02650533.2023.2207728

Pilling, M. D. (2022). *Queer and trans madness: Struggles for social justice*. Palgrave MacMillan. https://doi.org/10.1007/978-3-030-90413-5

Poole, J. (2011). *Behind the rhetoric: Mental health recovery in Ontario*. Fernwood Publishing.

Quiroz, B. D. R. V. (2022). A crazy, warrior and "respondona" Peruvian: All personal transformation is social and political. In P. Beresford and J. Russo (Eds.), *The Routledge international handbook of Mad Studies* (pp. 41–52). Routledge. https://doi.org/10.4324/9780429465444-6

Reaume, G. (2002). Lunatic to patient to person: Nomenclature in psychiatric history and the influence of patients' activism in North America. *International Journal of Law and Psychiatry*, 25(4), 405–426. https://doi.org/10.1016/S0160-2527(02)00130-9

Reaume, G. (2006). Mad people's history. *Radical History Review*, 2006(94), 170–182. https://doi.org/10.1215/01636545-2006-94-170

Reaume, G. (2008, July 14). A history of Psychiatric Survivor Pride Day during the 1990s. *The Consumer/Survivor Information Resource Centre Bulletin*, 374, 2–3.

Reaume, G. (2010). Psychiatric patient built wall tours at the Centre for Addiction and Mental Health (CAMH), Toronto, 2000–2010. *Left History: An Interdisciplinary Journal of Historical Inquiry and Debate*, 15(1). https://doi.org/10.25071/1913-9632.35828

Reaume, G. (2019). Creating Mad People's History as a university credit course since 2000. *New Horizons in Adult Education and Human Resource Development, 31*(1), 22–39. https://doi.org/10.1002/nha3.20238

Reaume, G. (2021). Mad activists and the left in Ontario, 1970s to 2000. In R. Ellis, S. Kendal, & S. J. Taylor (Eds.), *Voices in the history of madness: Personal and professional perspectives on mental health and illness* (pp. 307–332). Springer International Publishing. https://doi.org/10.1007/978-3-030-69559-0_15

Reaume, G. (2022). How is Mad Studies different from anti-psychiatry and critical psychiatry? In P. Beresford and J. Russo (Eds.), *The Routledge international handbook of Mad Studies* (pp. 98–107). Routledge. https://doi.org/10.4324/9780429465444-15

Reaume, G. (2024). The qualitative historical origins of Mad Studies in word and deed, 1436–1914. *Qualitative Inquiry.* https://doi.org/10.1177/10778004241253249

Reville, D. & Church, K. (2012). Mad activism enters its fifth decade: Psychiatric survivor organizing in Toronto. In A. Choudry, J. Hanley, & E. Shragge (Eds.), *Organize! Building from the local for global justice* (pp. 189–201). PM Press.

Reville, D. (2013). Is Mad Studies emerging as a new field of inquiry? In B. A. LeFrançois, R. Menzies, & G. Reaume, *Mad matters: A critical reader in Canadian Mad Studies* (pp. 170–180). Canadian Scholars Press.

Rimke, H. (2018). Sickening institutions: A feminist sociological analysis and critique of religion, medicine, and psychiatry. In J. Kilty & E. Dej (Eds.), *Containing madness: Gender and "psy" in institutional contexts* (pp. 15–39). Palgrave Macmillan. https://doi.org/10.1007/978-3-319-89749-3_2

Sapouna, L., & O'Donnell, A. (2017). "Madness" and activism in Ireland and Scotland, a dialogue. *Community Development Journal, 52*(3), 524–534. https://doi.org/10.1093/cdj/bsx031

Schalk, S. (2022). *Black disability politics*. Duke University Press. https://doi.org/10.1515/9781478027003

Schrader, S., Jones, N., & Shattell, M. (2013). Mad Pride: Reflections on sociopolitical identity and mental diversity in the context of culturally competent psychiatric care. *Issues in Mental Health Nursing*, *34*(1), 62–64. https://doi.org/10.3109/01612840.2012.740769

Shimrat, I. (1997). *Call me crazy: Stories from the Mad movement*. Press Gang Publishers.

Shimrat, I. (2018, August 16). *Resistance matters: The activism of Don Weitz*. Mad in America. www.madinamerica.com/2018/08/resistance-matters-activism-don-weitz/

Showalter, E. (1987). *The female malady*. Penguin Books.

Smith, D. E. & David, S. J. (1975). *Women look at psychiatry*. Press Gang Publishers.

Smith-Rosenberg, C. (1986). *Disorderly conduct: Visions of gender in Victorian America*. Oxford University Press.

Snyder, S. N., Pitt, K.-A., Shanouda, F., Voronka, J., Reid, J., & Landry, D. (2019). Unlearning through Mad Studies: disruptive pedagogical praxis. *Curriculum Inquiry*, *49*(4), 485–502. https://doi.org/10.1080/03626784.2019.1664254

Spandler, H. (2006). *Asylum to action: Paddington day hospital, therapeutic communities and beyond*. Jessica Kingsley Publishers.

Spandler, H. (2020). *Asylum*: A magazine for democratic psychiatry in England. In T. Burns & J. Foot (Eds.), *Basaglia's international legacy: From asylum to community* (pp 205–226). Oxford University Press. https://doi.org/10.1093/med/9780198841012.003.0013

Spandler, H., Anderson, J., & Sapey, B. (Eds.). (2015). *Madness, distress and the politics of disablement*. Policy Press. https://doi.org/10.1332/policypress/9781447314578.001.0001

Spandler, H. & Carr, S. (2021). A history of lesbian politics and the psy professions. *Feminism & Psychology*, *31*(1), 119–139. https://doi.org/10.1177/0959353520969297

Starkman, M. (2013) The movement. In B. A. LeFrançois, R. Menzies, & G. Reaume, *Mad matters: A critical reader in Canadian Mad Studies* (pp. 27–37). Canadian Scholars Press.

Stefan, H. C. (2018). A (head) case for a Mad humanities: Sula's Shadrack and Black madness. *Disability Studies Quarterly, 38*(4). https://doi.org/10.18061/dsq.v38i4.6378

Thorneycroft, R. (2020). Crip theory and Mad Studies: Intersections and points of departure. *Canadian Journal of Disability Studies, 9*(1), 91–121. https://doi.org/10.15353/cjds.v9i1.597

Ussher, J. M. (1991). *Women's madness: Misogyny or mental illness?* University of Massachusetts Press.

Ussher, J. M. (2011). *The madness of women.* Routledge. https://doi.org/10.4324/9780203806579

Voronka, J. (2019). Storytelling beyond the psychiatric gaze: Resisting resilience and recovery narratives. *Canadian Journal of Disability Studies, 8*(4), 8–30. https://doi.org/10.15353/cjds.v8i4.522

Walker, D. E. (2022). *Coyote's Swing: A memoir and critique of mental hygiene in Native America.* Washington State University Press.

Weitz, D. (2018). *Resistance matters: The radical vision of an antipsychiatry activist.* Mad in America. www.madinamerica.com/wp-content/uploads/2019/06/Resistance-Matters-April-2019.pdf

Wood, C. (2012, October 2). *Tales from the crip: This is what disability looks like.* Bitch Media (Library of Congress Web Archives). Retrieved from https://webarchive.loc.gov/all/20221124005013/https://www.bitchmedia.org/post/tales-from-the-crip-this-is-what-disability-looks-like-feminist-magazine-facebook-disabilities-visibility

Young, S. (2014, April). *I'm not your inspiration, thank you very much* [Video]. TEDxSydney. www.ted.com/talks/stella_young_i_m_not_your_inspiration_thank_you_very_much?utm_campaign=tedspread&utm_medium=referral&utm_source=tedcomshare

WHAT CAN MAD STUDIES HELP US UNDERSTAND?

There is no definition of Mad Studies on which everyone (or even all Mad activists and scholars) would agree. Mad Studies is multivalent, inter- and multi-disciplinary, and as such includes multiple perspectives across many academic disciplines (LeFrançois et al., 2013). Mad scholars and activists have emphasized the importance of keeping Mad Studies open, dynamic, and flexible (Costa, 2014; Gorman & LeFrançois, 2017). Perhaps the one thing that could be agreed upon about Mad Studies is that it is grounded in the knowledge of activists, Mad people, and those with lived experience of unjust institutions such as mental health, criminal justice, and immigration systems, and must remain accountable to these communities. As Gorman & LeFrançois (2017) put it, "mad studies takes place in a variety of spaces within or without academia, but never without community" (p. 108). Given the pluralistic, dynamic nature of Mad Studies, it does not seem possible or useful to provide a singular or proscriptive definition of Mad Studies. Therefore, this chapter does not define Mad Studies, nor does it provide an exhaustive account of the literature encompassing everything that has been created in the name of Mad Studies. Instead, it explores some answers to the question:

DOI: 10.4324/9781003561552-3

what can Mad Studies help us understand? Topics explored include the biomedical model of mental illness, the psy complex, madness, bodymind, Mad identity, sanism, epistemic injustice, and using a Mad lens to examine knowledge production.

THE BIOMEDICAL MODEL OF MENTAL ILLNESS AND THE PSY COMPLEX

Mad Studies helps us understand that the predominant way of conceptualizing and responding to madness and Mad people is based on a theoretical framework called the 'biomedical model of mental illness' and that this model should have no special status that places it above scrutiny and critique. The biomedical model is so ubiquitous that it is not generally thought of *as* a model with specific beliefs, values, and ideologies that are culturally and historically specific. Rather, it is positioned as common sense and the ultimate truth about madness, and anyone who has a different explanation is seen as misinformed, a conspiracy theorist, or Mad (Pilling et al, 2018; Ringer & Holen, 2016). Mad Studies exposes the biomedical model as a framework with underlying ideologies just like any other, and critiques and analyses the inherent injustices within it.

The biomedical model categorizes various experiences, behaviours, thoughts, and ways of being and thinking as indicative of individual biological pathologies that can be scientifically evidenced and universally applied. Mental illness is seen as a biological deficit that can be diagnosed according to a taxonomy of disorders that have "characteristic common features" (Lewis, 2006, p. 107). Biomedicalism locates the cause of mental illness in biological factors such as brain structure, genetics, and biochemistry and seeks to cure and treat it through means characterized as medical in nature (e.g. pharmaceuticals, electroshock). According to the biomedical model, there is a binary divide between the Mad and the sane. In other words, some people are Mad while others are sane, as opposed to madness and distress being seen as part of the human experience. The biomedical model is highly individualistic, locating the problem of, and the solution to, mental illness in the 'sick' individual who must be cured or treated through medical intervention. Rimke (2016) coined the term 'psychocentrism' in order to describe this individualistic approach as a form of injustice. She defines psychocentrism as the "view that human problems are due to a biologically based flaw or deficit in the bodies and/or minds of individual subjects. Psychocentrism is itself a form of social injustice, where individual reformation rather than social and economic justice is promoted" (Rimke, 2016, p. 5).

The individualism of the biomedical model is a hallmark of the neoliberal worldview that dominates countries in the Global North. In a neoliberal context, the logic of the market prevails and is applied to social institutions and policies resulting in less spending on social welfare. A key feature of neoliberalism is the downloading of collective responsibilities onto individuals. Neoliberalism emphasizes the need to find "private solutions to social problems" (Morrow, 2013, p. 328). As such, it is compatible with the biomedical model, in which understandings of, and solutions to, madness and distress are individualized.

The biomedical model has been exported from the Global North to the Global South in what has been called 'psychiatric imperialism' (Fernando, 2010; Mills, 2014). This exportation is a colonial project that has dismissed, undermined, and pathologized non-medicalized and Indigenous ways of understanding madness and distress in the Global South and characterized them as "harmful superstitions" that are the product of "backward" cultures (Timimi, 2011, p. 157). Pharmaceutical companies profit from such expansion, giving them a vested interest in the globalization of the biomedical model (Timimi, 2011).

The biomedical model underpins many disciplines. Psychiatry has positioned itself as a medical science and is therefore most obviously informed by biomedicalism, however, this perspective extends to psychology and beyond. As Rapley et al. (2011) state, "mainstream psychology ... while sometimes appearing to offer alternative approaches, essentially supports the positivist psychiatric project of codifying human suffering into disease-like categories" (p. 1). There are versions of psychiatry and psychology that place more emphasis on social context, but as Beresford (2005) claims, even these "have taken as given the over-arching medicalised framework of 'mental illness,' although differing in the extent to which they saw it as a consequence of nature or nurture" (p. 36). The same claim has been made about social work practice and education (Poole et al., 2012).

Mad Studies scholars have named the massive proliferation of the biomedical model the 'psy complex.' Rimke (2016) defines the psy complex as:

A hegemonic formation comprised of a loosely defined group of experts connected through their professional and social status, particularly psychiatrists, psychologists, psychiatric nurses, psychotherapists, psychoanalysts, and social workers. It is conceived as a heterogeneous network of agents, sites, practices, products and techniques for the production, dissemination, legitimation, and utilization of psy truths.

(p. 4)

While the prefix 'psy' is meant to capture its origins in psychiatry and psychology, the word 'complex' is used to indicate that biomedical beliefs and practices extend well beyond medical settings such as hospitals and doctor's offices to infiltrate institutions, policy (e.g. mental health strategies, social assistance regulations), services (e.g. community organizations, private therapists), industry (e.g. pharmaceutical industry), education (e.g. post-secondary campuses, research funding bodies), popular culture (e.g. news media, movies), means of creating and disseminating information (e.g. anti-stigma campaigns, academic research), and even groups for people with lived experience (e.g. some patient-rights groups).

The extensive reach of the psy complex has facilitated widespread investment in the idea that madness and distress are due to malfunctioning brains and must be responded to as such

(LeFrançois et al., 2016). This makes the biomedical model re-markably resilient to critique. Despite years of well-funded re-search, there is no conclusive evidence that proves the scientific validity of the concept of mental disorder as something that is objectively verifiable through scientific or medical testing or distinct biomarkers (Boyle, 2011; Burstow, 2015; Fernando, 2017; LeFrançois & Voronka, 2022; Rimke, 2016; Whitaker, 2001). And yet, this is a highly controversial, perhaps even in-flammatory observation, because of the dominance of the bio-medical model via the psy complex. The work of Mad Studies scholars and activists in naming the psy complex and identify-ing its effects will continue to be crucial in undoing its power to operate as an unmarked norm that cannot be questioned. Part of this work is also in proffering different explanations of the nature of madness.

WHAT IS MADNESS?

Mad Studies demands that we find different answers to the very meaning of the beliefs, behaviours, and bodymind experiences that are currently characterized as being indicative of mental ill-ness and falling under the purview of mental health practition-ers, policies, and systems. As discussed, the predominant way of understanding these experiences is through the biomedical model, which positions them as various forms of mental illness, explained by individual deficits such as faulty brain chemistry and genetics. In contrast, Mad Studies historicizes madness, or in other words, places it within its historical context, acknowl-edging that it has only been since the 19th century that madness has been understood as a medical issue in the Global North (Rimke & Hunt, 2002). For example, in the 1600s, European cultures that espoused Christianity viewed madness through a religious lens, as demonic possession and the work of Satan (Porter, 2002). In the 19th century, Tibetan ways of under-standing madness "combined the teachings of orthodox Bud-dhism" with concepts of "herbal therapy and diet derived from Ayurveda ... to form a method of person-centred treatment" (Fernando, 2017, p. 32). The 'healthification' of madness (i.e. seeing madness as a matter of health) is "a conflation that is particular to Western culture but one that is increasingly being spread worldwide as local non-Western systems are being globalized" (Fernando, 2017, p. 20). Mad Studies points to the ways in which understandings of madness shift across time and according to context and culture, though it has often done so in a Eurocentric fashion (Joseph, 2015). Mad Studies also allows us to see that madness should not be reduced to distress. There are times when madness takes the form of distress, or when it is experienced as very distressing. There are also times when madness is experienced as pleasurable, productive, creative, spiritual, transcendental, sacred, or simply neutral.

Mad Studies takes various approaches to understanding madness and distress as social, and as inextricable from the dominant culture(s) in which we are immersed. As Gorman (2013) states, "Mad Studies takes social, relational, identity-based, and anti-oppression approaches to questions of mental/psychological/behavioural difference, and is articulated, in part, against an analytic of mental illness" (p. 269). Gorman's definition is likely purposely broad to indicate that there is no firm consensus within Mad Studies as to the origins and reasons for madness, or even that such explanation is necessary. Similar to those who resist the heterosexist compulsion to explain the origins of queerness, we could simply accept that madness is a natural and expected part of human existence and leave it at that. However, Gorman's positioning of Mad Studies as being "against an analytic of mental illness" (at least "in part") is key. Much of Mad Studies' conceptualizations of madness have been articulated against, and in resistance to, psy-based definitions of mental illness. In other words, madness has often been characterized variously by Mad scholars and activists in terms of what it is *not*; for example, as not pathological, not an illness, not a deficit, not biological, not medical, and not necessarily in need of curing. It makes sense that Mad Studies has conceptualized madness in contradistinction to the biomedical model, because this model is so predominant as to invoke "downright hostility" towards those who dare to resist it or theorize Mad alternatives (Menzies et al., 2013, p. 11).

SOCIAL VERSUS BIOLOGICAL FACTORS

As the above suggests, one key difference between the way that madness is conceptualized within the biomedical model and how it is understood by Mad Studies is the extent to which the biological (e.g. brain chemistry, genetics, hormones) and the social (e.g. housing and food insecurity, structural oppression, experiences of trauma) shape and create experiences of madness and distress.

There are some shared understandings amongst Mad scholars and activists about the relationship between madness and the social; for example, most (or dare I say all) would agree that experiences of oppression such as poverty, racism, and transphobia cause distress and can be 'maddening.' However, Mad scholars and activists cannot be said to be united in their position on the relationship between madness, the social, and the biological. There is space within Mad Studies for varying positions on the matter; there is no need for a unified explanation of madness, though some may disagree that this is unnecessary (Beresford & Rose, 2023).

The relationship between Mad Studies and understandings of madness as biological and/or social can be explained as follows. For a moment, think of the various explanations of madness on a continuum, with the biological (our behaviours, experiences, and interests are biologically determined) on one end, and the social (human characteristics are determined by the environment, culture, and context) on the other, and many shades of grey in between. This is one possible way of understanding Mad Studies' various conceptualizations of madness in relation to biological and social factors.[1] However, the problem with a continuum is that it relies on a binary (social/biological) even while acknowledging shades of grey in the middle. It also does not fully account for understandings of madness as spiritual, religious, or as something that is not fully captured by its relationship to the social or biological. The exclusion of the spiritual is one means of marginalizing Indigenous, Black, racialized, and queer understandings of madness (Cuthand, n.d.; Dwornik, 2021; Ezell, 2019; Jackson, 2002; Johnk,

2021; Lavallée, 2021; Lavallée, 2022; Lavallée & Poole, 2010; Linklater, 2014; Persaud, 2022). Perhaps it is better to think of madness as a constellation with as many explanations for it as there are stars in the sky, variously placed within the galaxy of Mad Studies.[2] These could be social, cultural, relational, discursive, religious, spiritual, experiential, transcendental, biological, or some combination thereof that eschews a social/biological binary altogether.

That said, it is important to acknowledge that, as explained in Chapter 1, Mad Studies leans heavily towards the social due to its roots in the social model of disability and activist resistance to medical oppression and iatrogenic harms. It is also important to note that the various stars in the galaxy are not value-neutral; some hold more cultural weight than others. Explanations of madness and distress that incorporate the biological are seen as more legitimate within dominant discourses due to their proximity to the biomedical model (Rimke, 2018). The explanations of madness that are least palatable within the mainstream are grounded in strong critiques of colonialism, capitalism, cisheteropatriarchy, and white supremacy. These explanations are also the hardest to articulate without being dismissed as being too radical or on the "lunatic fringe" (Pilling, 2022, p. 29).

Mad Studies scholars and activists who argue that madness is inherently social and relational are often wrongly accused of claiming that experiences of distress and madness do not exist or are not real. This is particularly true of Mad Studies scholars and activists who believe that it can be unhelpful to medicalize madness, that is, to treat it as a medical issue in need of psychiatric intervention. This speaks to the extent to which biological explanations have a stranglehold on what is considered real and authentic, even though there are many social constructs (such as time and money) that are clearly real in that they dictate many aspects of our lives and have significant material consequences. Queer Studies scholars have shown that sexuality and gender are real even though they are not based in biology. In other words, there is no gay gene nor is there a biologically based male/female binary (Butler, 2004; Fausto-Sterling, 2000) but that does not mean that queer, heterosexual, trans, and cisgender people do not exist. Like madness, the ways that humans understand sexuality and gender change according to culture and across historical contexts, and it follows that these shifting social constructs are not biological. And yet, sexuality and gender are real, and society is organized around these concepts in such a way as to have material consequences. Likewise, madness does not have to be caused by biological factors to be real.

DOING AWAY WITH BINARIES: BODYMIND

Now that I have explained the social/biological binary, I propose that binary thinking is not terribly useful, and explore the Mad Studies concept of bodymind as a promising example of non-binary theorizing about madness. It can be difficult to fully divest from the social/biological binary in meaning-making about madness because the use of this binary is not just restricted to debates about the nature of madness. Binary thinking is a core element of Western, colonial knowledge production and as such it is widely used to debate the origins of many human characteristics such as race, sex, gender, and sexuality. For example, queer theorists, feminists, and gender scholars have long struggled with the thorny issues presented by the social/biological binary when it comes to explaining the nature of gender, sex, and sexuality. Some, like Anne Fausto-Sterling (2000), have encouraged scholars to move away from the social/biological binary. She explores the promise of developmental systems theory (DST) for doing away with binary thinking (or as she puts it, the nature vs nurture binary) when it comes to understanding sex, gender, and sexuality. She explains that DST rejects the idea that there are two distinct types of processes, "one guided by genes, hormones, and brain cells (that is, nature), and the other by the environment, experience, learning, and inchoate social forces (that is, nurture)" (p. 25). She provides an example from the work of a DST theorist, Peter Taylor, about "a goat born with no front legs" that developed an "S-shaped spine" similar to a human spine due to the way it walked on its hind legs throughout its life. As she states, "neither its genes nor its environment determined its anatomy. Only the ensemble had such power" (p. 26). Fausto-Sterling uses such frameworks to dissect binaries such as the argument that sex is biological while gender is social. She shows how *both* sex and gender are constructed and yet, like the goat with two legs, our bodies are "made of materials" that are immersed within, and created through, our social contexts (p. 28).

Taking a look at the debates about the social/biological binary that have taken place in like-minded and overlapping subject areas such as Gender Studies and queer theory can be useful. It is helpful to look at Fausto-Sterling's work as an example of the importance of moving away from binary thinking. As a relatively new field, Mad Studies can learn from these debates and think through their application to Mad Studies rather than simply repeating them. As Mad Studies continues to grow, Mad theory about the nature of madness will no doubt develop and become more fully and mindfully articulated. It will be unhelpful to become caught up in binary frameworks. As Fausto-Sterling (2000) cautions, "Politically, the nature/nurture framework holds enormous dangers. Although some hope that a belief in the nature side of things will lead to greater tolerance, past history suggests that the opposite is also possible" (p. 26).

In some ways Price's (2011, 2015) conceptualization of 'bodymind' is reminiscent of Fausto-Sterling's (2000) explanation of the goat with two legs and can be seen as an example of a Mad Studies concept that eschews binary thinking by rejecting both the social/biological binary and the mind/body binary. Price (2015) mobilizes the concept of 'bodymind' as "a materialist feminist DS [Disability Studies] concept" (p. 270) that challenges the colonial Cartesian dualism that positions the body as distinct from the mind.[3] The term 'bodymind' is used to indicate not just that the body and mind cannot be separated, but that this single entity is emersed and created within sociopolitical contexts where the corporeal meets the environment in multi-directional encounters in which the bodymind is in a constant state of becoming (Price, 2015). As Price puts it, the bodymind is "a socio politically constituted and material entity that emerges through both structural (power and violence-laden) contexts and also individual (specific) experience" (p. 271). Elsewhere, Price (2011) jokes that "if it weren't so unwieldy" she "would be tempted to use something like psychobiosocialpoliticalbodymind" instead of 'bodymind' (p. 240). As this indicates, the concept of 'bodymind' eschews the mind/body dualism at the heart of the biomedical model, but it also destroys the social/biological binary that would position madness as *either* biological *or* social (or even somewhere in between).

The concept of 'bodymind' can be especially helpful for thinking through the relationship between madness and structural oppression such as transphobia, homophobia, and racism because oppression shapes our bodily experience. For example, if one is living in poverty (a form of structural oppression) without regular access to food, this in turn shapes one's bodily experience and wellness in a way that cannot easily be separated into the physical versus the mental or the biological versus the social. This is perhaps a more obvious example because of the tangible factor involved (i.e., food). However, all forms of oppression, including those that are intangible, can have detrimental effects on our bodyminds.

Following Price (2011, 2015), Schalk (2018) employs the concept of 'bodymind' in her work on Black women's speculative fiction. As Schalk notes, racism impacts wellbeing and the term 'bodymind' can highlight this: "As more research reveals the ways experiences and histories of oppression impact us mentally, physically, and even on a cellular level, the term bodymind can help highlight the relationship of nonphysical experiences of oppression – psychic stress – and overall well-being" (pp. 5–6). Schalk (2018) explains that the concept of 'bodymind' is particularly apt for discussions of racism, since the rejection of the mind/body dualism has a long history in communities of colour and amongst women, who have "challenged their association with pure embodiment and the degradation of the body as unable to produce knowledge" (p. 6).

As the work of Price and Schalk demonstrates, the Mad Studies concept of bodymind is a helpful way of thinking about madness that does not get caught up in fruitless debates about binaries. The way that madness gets conceptualized matters deeply because our understandings of madness shape how we respond to it, both individually and collectively as a society. The social/biological binary very much informs what is seen as important and fundable when it comes to responding to madness and distress. Will Landback, affordable housing, fair wages for all, and gender affirming care be seen as deeply intertwined with our collective wellbeing and 'mental health'? Or will millions more dollars be poured into the search for a biological basis for mental illness and funding psychiatric lockups to detain those who are struggling with the world we have created?

MAD IDENTITY

Mad Studies and activism provide the tools for self-understanding, for redefining experiences of madness, and for reclaiming a devalued identity. For some, identifying as 'Mad' can be a matter of pride and empowerment, and can be part of wresting one's bodymind from the clutches of the psy complex. Similar to reclamations of the word 'queer,' those who self-identify as Mad are taking a term that has been used to denigrate and diminish and are reclaiming it in a way that feels empowering. This use of 'Mad' as an identity turns the deficit model on its head, talking back to the psy complex that has long positioned Mad people as defective. Taking on the term 'Mad' can indicate opposition to being eclipsed by the imposed designation of 'patient' and can signal agency, awareness, and connection to Mad history and knowledge. Like 'queer,' the term 'Mad' is a term that connotes resistance to hegemonic norms and connection to politicized collectives and communities (Spandler, 2017; Spandler & Barker, 2016; Pilling, 2022).

'Mad' can be used as an umbrella term to include the various ways in which people may self-identify including (but not limited to) service user, consumer, person with lived experience, psychiatric survivor, ex-patient, and ex-inmate (Diamond, 2013). The acronym c/s/x includes consumer, survivor, and ex-patient and is sometimes used in place of 'Mad' when a more specific term is needed. Like 'queer,' Mad is a flexible, dynamic, contestatory term that means different things to different people. 'Mad' is not meant to indicate a singular or "essentialized identity category" (Spandler & Poursanidou, 2019, p. 4). What unites some Mad people is sanist oppression under the psy complex, not an essentialized notion of what it means to be Mad (Diamond, 2013). However, as Joseph (2019) points out, "racialized and indigenous peoples often find themselves at the mercy of criminal justice and immigration systems, while mental health services are differentially accessed or imposed" (p. 1). Defining Mad identity as having lived experience of the mental health system is white-centric and erases the lived realities of Black, Indigenous, and people of colour (Pattadath, 2016).

As this indicates, Mad identity and politics struggle with essentialism, or in other words, the notion that there is, or should be, a unified and clearly defined set of characteristics that define Mad identity and describes a certain type of person and politics. As Voronka (2016) cautions, falling prey to essentialism results in "whitewashing how madness lands and is graphed on bodies differently" (p. 197). Sanism operates in tandem with other systems of power such as white supremacy and cisheteropatriarchy and thus impacts people differently depending on context and social location (Abdillahi et al., 2017; Gorman et al., 2013; Meerai et al., 2016). Mad Studies and activism must remain vigilant against creating "a singular and essentialized story of the experiences of mad people, mad communities, and mad cultural production" (LeFrançois & Voronka, 2022, p. 118).

Relatedly, not everyone who has a mental illness label imposed on them takes on a Mad identity. While some may have never heard of it, others overtly reject it for various reasons, including varying degrees of investment in the biomedical model, discomfort with a term that has been used in discriminatory ways, lack of affective connection with the term (i.e. it doesn't feel like 'home'), or lack of experiences of oppression within mental health systems (whether through deliberate avoidance and/or privilege). Some service users believe that the term 'Mad' romanticizes distress, is too unclear, or divisive (Beresford, 2020).

For some members of marginalized groups such as queer and trans people and Black, Indigenous, and people of colour, the term 'Mad' may not resonate because other identities (for example as trans, or as Indigenous) are more central, or because it is risky to take on yet another marginalized identity (Diamond, 2013; Pilling, 2022). For some who have been maddened or disabled by racism, colonialism, transphobia, poverty, and other forms of oppression, taking on a Mad or disabled identity may not feel empowering or prideful (Deerinwater et al., 2023; Schalk, 2022). Likewise, those whose identities have been, or continue to be, conflated with mental illness and madness (for example, Black and/or 2SLGBTQI people) may not identify with the term 'Mad' (Doharty, 2024; Pilling, 2022). Further, Mad politics and identity can be alienating because it has not realized a truly intersectional politic, for example, by incorporating a fulsome understanding of colonialism and decolonization (Dwornik, 2021; Joseph, 2015) or of transphobia and cisnormativity (Cosantino & Pilling, 2024; Pilling, 2022, forthcoming).

It is important to understand that a refusal of the moniker 'Mad' does not necessarily indicate a rejection of Mad Studies, politics, and activism (though it may). It is possible to experience madness, and/or oppression under the psy complex and not self-identify as Mad, but be very much aligned with, and participate in, Mad scholarship and activism. There are also those who are more clearly positioned as allies (those without lived experience of madness or psychiatrization) but who are personally and politically invested in Mad Studies and activism (Spandler & Poursanidou, 2019). Conversely, the adoption of

Mad as an identity does not necessarily indicate wholesale rejection of the biomedical model and all psychiatric services. There are those who identify as Mad who must, or who want to, make use of psychiatric services. As explained throughout this book, binaries (including pro/anti psychiatry) are unhelpful and do not reflect the nuanced realities of people's lives. Mad Studies and activism are complex enough to have space for a multiplicity of identities and subject positions in relation to, or outside of, the psy complex.

SANISM AND EPISTEMIC INJUSTICE

Mad Studies advances sanism as an analytic that sheds light on the oppression of Mad people and the way madness is perceived. The term was coined by Birnbaum (1960) but was introduced into broader use by Perlin (1992) and has since become central to Mad Studies (Poole et al., 2012). Sanism is a form of systemic marginalization and exploitation that is analogous to, intersects with, and is co-constitutive of, other kinds of oppression such as ableism, racism, transphobia, homophobia, classism, and sexism. Sanism, like all forms of oppression, manifests at the cultural, structural, and interpersonal levels. It is multi-layered and reflects an intricate web of beliefs and practices that position Mad people (and those deemed as such) as less human than those seen as sane. As this also indicates, sanism relies on a binary that assumes that some of us are Mad and some of us are sane, and that those who are Mad are inferior to those who are sane.

Sanism is different from the more mainstream concept of 'stigma,' which is ideologically tied to biomedicalism and is widely used to name prejudicial beliefs and discrimination against 'the mentally ill.'[4] Sanism possesses more "robust explanatory power than stigma" and

> accounts for both discrimination against those perceived as mad *and* for psychiatric violence, while 'stigma' only accounts for the former. Indeed, in contemporary mental

health campaigns, the 'problem' with stigma is that it causes delays in 'getting help' from what are, ultimately, oppressive systems.
(Gorman & LeFrançois, 2017, p. 110, emphasis added)

Analyses of stigma often stay at the individual level, positioning it as prejudicial beliefs harboured by some individuals that can be countered through the inclusion of those 'struggling with mental health issues' and more widespread acceptance of the idea that there is no shame in 'mental illness.' This is often linked to the idea that mental illness is a biological deficiency, and therefore the mentally ill cannot help it, should not be blamed for it, and must not be hindered from seeking treatment for it from mental health services. Whether individual or systemic, analyses of stigma do not expose the oppression and violence embedded within biomedicalism and inflicted by psychiatric systems. Stigma is therefore a concept that can be used to further the psy complex, rather than to limit, critique, or abolish it. Sanism is thus an important analytical contribution of Mad Studies and must be understood as being distinct from the concept of stigma.

Sanism is inextricably bound up with the concept of epistemic injustice (Fricker, 2007). Leblanc and Kinsella's (2016) influential application of the concept of epistemic injustice to sanism and the Mad community explains that sanism and epistemic injustice are interrelated. Following Fricker (2007, 2010) they define epistemic injustice as taking place "when a person is insulted or wronged in their capacity as knower" (Leblanc & Kinsella, 2016, p. 61). Epistemic injustice discredits, subjugates, and denies the humanity of Mad people, or as they state, "If it is our ability to *know* that makes us distinctively human … it is no wonder that the 'powerful' have historically undermined, insulted, or otherwise wronged the 'powerless' in this capacity, as a means for denouncing their humanity" (Leblanc & Kinsella, 2016, p. 61). A salient feature of sanism is the assumption that those deemed Mad cannot be trusted to have an accurate representation of reality, including (or perhaps especially) regarding their own experience and bodymind. As Liegghio (2013) puts it, sanism dictates that Mad people have "a flawed or disordered way of seeing, perceiving, judging, and thus, knowing reality" (p. 126). In this way, epistemic injustice is committed against Mad people, who are denied the status of "legitimate knowers with legitimate knowledge and ways of being" (Liegghio, 2013, p. 129).

Psychiatric violence and the contravention of Mad people's rights is often a manifestation of epistemic injustice, facilitated by sanism. Mad people's assumed inability to participate in a shared, socially accepted reality and know their own bodyminds is used as justification for infringement on their bodily autonomy and capacity to make personal decisions about their lives, finances, and medical treatment. For example, psychiatric constructs such as 'insight' have been used to enact epistemic injustice by invalidating Mad people's perceived capacity to know their own experience and thereby make decisions about their bodyminds (Hamilton & Roper, 2006; Leblanc & Kinsella, 2016; Pilling et al., 2018). Mad people who attempt to refuse biomedical treatments and explanations of their madness are often characterized as lacking insight into their illness, thereby invalidating their resistance and their status as 'legitimate knowers' (Galasiński & Ziółkowska, 2013; Høyer, 2000; Pilling et al., 2018). Likewise, Mad people who wish to contest involuntary hospitalization, forced drugging, and electroshock have little recourse in court because they are defined as unreliable narrators who lack insight, whereas the physician is seen as the expert or 'legitimate knower' who knows what is best for the patient (Diesfeld & Sjöström, 2007; Pilling et al., 2018). These issues are compounded for queer, trans, Black, Indigenous, and people of colour, who are even more likely to be seen as lacking insight (Pilling et al., 2018). This is epistemic injustice and sanism in action.

Sanism is normalized and widely accepted as a matter of common sense. It is ubiquitous and is often used as a catch-all for unpopular or socially disruptive behaviour and beliefs. Consider, for example, how often politicians are characterized as 'crazy,' 'mentally ill,' 'psychopathic,' 'sociopathic,' and as having a 'disordered personality.' This is sanism at work; the unpopular and sometimes violent policies and beliefs espoused by various politicians are characterized as undesirable or beyond reason and thereby associated with madness rather than being seen for what they are; a reflection of contemporary cultural values. Politicians and their ideas do not exist in a vacuum, rather, they reflect elements of ideologies and values shared by enough people to get them elected (see also Bruce, 2021, p. 28). This is why removing one oppressive politician from office will not get rid of the problem. In other words, the problem is not one individual politician's supposed madness; the problem is the widespread social values that enable and perpetuate structural oppression.

Relatedly, sanism positions Mad people as violent and dangerous. This sanist belief is heightened when it comes to violence that is characterized as being particularly heinous. For example, consider how frequently those who commit such crimes are immediately characterized as Mad in the media and in mainstream discourse. Sanism makes it possible to believe that sane people do not have the capacity to commit odious or 'extreme' forms of violence, especially if they are white, even though history and current conditions show evidence of mass acceptance of violent, exploitative, and murderous ideologies and practices among white people (for example colonialism, chattel slavery, and Naziism). The ideologies of white supremacy dictate that it is people of colour and Indigenous people who are 'innately' violent, and so acts of heinous violence committed by white people are recast as mental illness as a means of distancing and turning away from our collective responsibility to address the underlying cause of such violence (for example, white supremacy, anti-Indigeneity, anti-Black racism, and antisemitism). This is just one way in which sanism is bound up with other forms of oppression; it is mobilized to individualize acts of white violence and deny the cultural context in which they occur. In other words, madness is a convenient scapegoat that individualizes the problem and ignores the larger picture. And yet, because Indigenous, Black, and racialized people are always already positioned as dangerous and potentially violent, they tend to bear the brunt of the resulting fearmongering about Mad people as dangerous. As Joseph (2019) states, "when dangerousness is assumed, tropes of incivility, savagery, and madness are often relied upon to distance, dehumanize, and delegitimize the lived experiences of racialized people and indigenous people" (p. 11). The sanist belief that Mad people are dangerous is used to justify psychiatric violence and coercive control of Mad lives and bodyminds, especially when it comes to queer, trans, Black, Indigenous, and Mad people of colour (Abdillahi et al., 2017; Joseph 2014, 2019; Meerai et al., 2016; Mannoe, 2023; Pilling, 2022).

As this indicates, sanism is racialized, or as Meerai et al. (2016) state, "sanism exists on a continuum depending on privilege, and it is always and especially compounded when it is visited on racialized bodies" (p. 22). In particular, the combination of anti-Black racism and sanism known as anti-Black sanism positions Mad Black people as especially threatening, dangerous, in need of management, and incapable of knowing their own experiences and bodyminds (Abdillahi et al., 2017; Meerai et al., 2016; Pilling, 2021). Abdillahi, Meerai, and Poole (2016, 2017) coined the term 'anti-Black sanism' to describe this form of oppression and to explicate its wide-ranging impacts. Their work has been crucial in illuminating how anti-Black sanism permeates mental health systems when it comes to "communication, diagnosis, hospitalization, treatment, intervention, and the involvement of the criminal justice system" (Abdillahi et al., 2017, p. 122). Anti-Black sanism gives name to injustices experienced by Black people, including the disproportionate use of coercive referrals and carceral treatment such as seclusion and mechanical and chemical restraint (Knight et al., 2022) and the disproportionate diagnosing of Black men with schizophrenia, a phenomenon that has its roots in the pathologizing and undermining of civil rights resistance (Metzl, 2009).

Anti-Black sanism is not limited to the workings of mental health systems; it also shapes interactions between police and

Black Mad people, with many such encounters having violent and deadly consequences for Black people (Mannoe, 2023; Meerai, Abdillahi, & Poole, 2016) and inflicting collective trauma on Black communities (Waldron, 2021). For example, police responses to mental health-related calls resulted in death for Black Ontarians Andrew Loku, Regis Korchinski-Paquet, D'Andre Campbell, and Ejaz Choudry (Nasser, 2020a; Nasser, 2023). Likewise, a Black, trans woman died after being taken into custody by police under the auspices of Ontario's Mental Health Act in 2020. The circumstances of her death have yet to be explained, and she was misgendered by Ontario's Special Investigation Unit in press releases about the incident (Nasser, 2020b).

In sum, sanism is a mechanism through which Mad people are subjugated, controlled, and (mis)represented within the cultural imaginary, with dire consequences including infringement on autonomy and agency, violence, and in some cases, even death. The impact of sanism has disproportionate effects depending on subject position and social location. In other words, Mad people who are also Indigenous, Black, racialized, queer, trans, poor, or otherwise multiply oppressed will bear the harshest outcomes of sanism.

UNDERSTANDING KNOWLEDGE PRODUCTION THROUGH A MAD LENS

Employing a Mad lens can mean more than one thing. In this section, I explain how a Mad lens can be used to critically examine processes of knowledge production and how medical and scientific knowledge has been weaponized against Mad people. In Chapter 3, I discuss how Mad Studies is itself a form of knowledge production. In other words, this section focuses on employing a Mad lens as a means of *understanding* and *examining* knowledge production while Chapter 3 focuses on using a Mad lens as a means of *creating* knowledge, while recognizing that these are very much intertwined.

The creation of academic knowledge is not a neutral, a-political set of discoveries based on objective observations by disinterested parties. The foundation of most (if not all) of the medical and scientific knowledge that we rely on today rests on the violent exploitation of marginalized groups. Much of this knowledge was created for the benefit of white people at the expense of Black, Indigenous, and people of colour and in the process inflicted great pain and suffering on these groups (Schalk, 2022, p. 65). If you need further evidence of this, take a look at the history of gynecology and the excruciating unanesthetized experimental surgeries conducted on enslaved Black women without consent (Ojanuga, 1993; Washington, 2006) or the nutrition experiments conducted on Indigenous children in Canadian residential schools (Mosby, 2013). Coloniality, anti-Blackness, and white supremacy lie at the heart of Western medicine and science (and the rest of academic knowledge production). The psy disciplines that have produced much of what is accepted as truth about madness are no different and are entangled with the history of science and medicine (Howell, 2018).

Mad Studies can help us reexamine who creates knowledge and how, with whose interests in mind, and with whose bodies on the line. A Mad Studies lens can illuminate how medicine and science have interpellated, or brought certain subjects into being, in ways that have justified their exploitation, that is, as inverts, degenerates, lunatics, imbeciles, and idiots suffering from feeble-mindedness; or, in a word, 'defectives.' There are sanist and ableist medical histories attached to each one of these terms (see Reaume, 2002), and they have also been weaponized against queer and trans people as well as Black, Indigenous, and people of colour in ways that show us that sanism and ableism are mutually constitutive with white supremacy, cisheteronormativity, and other systems of power (Clare, 2019). Mad Studies sheds light on the harms perpetrated against Mad people that have been justified and legitimized through scientific and medical knowledge production in the past, and their ongoing legacies in the present. These harms have been accomplished through dehumanizing those deemed undesirable and inferior by creating pathologizing knowledge about them that positions them as defective, a concept that is inherently ableist (Clare, 2019). Clare (2019) asks,

> Across the centuries, how many communities have been declared inherently defective by white people, rich people, nondisabled people, men backed by medical, scientific, academic, and state authority? I ask this question rather than answer it, because any list I create will be incomplete.
>
> (p. 3)

Clare (2019) gives some examples of the many groups whose bodyminds have been labelled defective as a way of justifying their exploitation, including enslaved Black Africans, immigrants refused entry to the United States at Ellis Island, lesbians and gay men subjected to conversion therapy, and white women suffragists (p. 3). Notions of disability and madness have long been used to characterize various marginalized groups as 'defective' as a means of legitimizing violence and genocide, demonstrating that white supremacy and cisheteropatriarchy are often articulated through sanism and ableism. Clare (2019) explains that,

> Defectiveness holds such power because ableism builds and maintains the very notion that defective body-minds are bad, undesirable, disposable.... Any person or community named defective can be targeted without question or hesitation for eradication, imprisonment, institutionalization. The ableist invention of defectiveness unequivocally names many body- minds wrong.
>
> (p. 3)

An oft used historical example that illustrates the mutually constitutive nature of racism, white supremacy, and sanism in the creation of psy knowledge is the work of Samuel Cartwright and the diagnoses he created to justify slavery and white violence in the 1800s. Cartwright invented a condition called 'drapetomania' to pathologize enslaved people who tried to escape (Clare, 2019; Fernando, 2010; Gilman, 1985; Jackson, 2002). This diagnosis reflected, and served to justify, the dominant white supremacist narrative that enslavement was the natural condition for Black people and so the behaviour of trying to escape enslavement was pathologized as disordered behaviour due to mental illness. Likewise, Cartwright's 'dysaesthesia aethiopis' was said to affect those who had been enslaved and would cause them to destroy property and create social disorder without white violence to keep them in check (Fernando, 2010). A more recent example of the confluence of racism, white supremacy, and sanism is knowledge production regarding schizophrenia (Fernando, 2010; Metzl, 2009). Metzl (2009) shows how during the civil rights era, schizophrenia changed from being "an illness of white feminine docility to one of Black male hostility from a confluence of social and medical forces" (p. xv). As Fernando (2010) also argues, "political, social and ideological pressures" shape diagnosis, and prevalent racist ideas about Black people (for example as dangerous) can result in the pathologizing of Black people and Black life (p. 68).

These examples should not be seen as isolated, or as the product of a few 'bad apple' scientists who happened to be racist. Rather, it needs to be understood that the development of "the general field of Western knowledge" (including psychiatry and psychology) in the 19th century relied upon deeply racist values from the Enlightenment period (Fernando, 2017, p. 21). As Bruce (2021) states, the Age of Enlightenment made concepts of reason and rationality "essential for achieving modern personhood, joining civil society, and participating in liberal politics" (p. 4). As he goes on to argue, only white men were positioned as having the capacity for reason:

Reason has been entangled, from those very Enlightenment roots, with misogynist, colonialist, ableist, antiblack, and other pernicious ideologies. The fact is that female people, indigenous people, colonized people, neurodivergent people, and black people have all been violently excluded from the edifice of Enlightenment Reason - with reasonable doctrines justifying those exclusions.

(p. 4)

Psychiatry and psychology emerged in combination with race science, which created racial taxonomies and hierarchies of intelligence placing white people at the top (Fernando, 2017, p. 19). Racialized peoples and cultures were characterized as uncivilized, primitive, and biologically inferior to white Europeans and Americans (Fernando, 2010, 2017).

Psychiatry and psychology have been used as tools of colonial violence (Harper, 1988; Joseph, 2019; Kanani, 2011). Since the inception of the psy disciplines, knowledge production about Indigenous peoples and cultures created by non-Indigenous scholars characterized them as primitive, inferior, and underdeveloped (Waldram, 2004). Racist knowledge production within the psy disciplines justified the involuntary institutionalization of Indigenous people in psychiatric institutions, facilitating colonial land theft (Kanani, 2011; Menzies & Palys, 2006, Yellow Bird, 2004; Walker, 2022). Indigenous writers have shown how incarceration in psychiatric institutions was a form of colonial social control masquerading as treatment (Harper, 1988; Walker, 2022; Yellow Bird, 2004). Colonial ideologies continue to underpin mental health care practice (Lavallée & Poole, 2010; Nelson, 2012). Indigenous people are still overrepresented in psychiatric systems (Voronka & LeFrançois, 2022) and current mental health care services "continue colonial relations and projects" (Joseph, 2019, p. 8). Disproportionately high suicide rates amongst Indigenous peoples are explained as a matter of defective genetics, or as Chrisjohn et al. (2017) state, "another aspect of our general sub-humanity" rather than the result of genocidal conditions created by colonialism (p. 41).

The medical history of regulating and disciplining normative sexuality and gender is likewise tied up with notions of defectiveness (i.e. ableism and sanism) and has a shared history with race science. A clear example of this is the invention of 'inversion' as mental and physical illness, which was a concept theorized by sexologists in the late 1800s and early 1900s to pathologize the bodyminds of those not easily understood through prevailing cultural notions of normative gender and sexuality. In today's terminology, such people would perhaps be understood as queer, trans, and non-binary. Sexology also relied upon concepts central to race science, indicating the imbrication of racism, queer/transphobia, ableism, and sanism (Somerville, 2000; Pilling, 2022). The legacies of these ideas continue to shape practices within mental health services. As I have demonstrated elsewhere through analyses of inpatient psychiatric charts (Pilling, 2022), trans and non-binary people are still positioned as abject and bizarre within the normative psychiatric institution, especially those who are also transfeminine and/or Black, Indigenous, and people of colour. While trans and queer people feel the harshest effects of the gender/sexual norms that are violently enforced through the psy complex, these norms also affect cisgender and heterosexual people. They too are expected to live up to normative gendered/sexualized standards or else risk being seen and treated as disordered (Daley, 2021; Metzl et al., 2016). As Tosh (2017) states, "the concept of normality has become so constrained that it represents an idealized form of white, middle class, heterosexual, cisgender masculinity that is impossible to attain" (p. 263).

In sum, Mad Studies can help us understand that the creation of medical and scientific knowledge is inextricable from the worldviews and context in which it is created and has lasting impacts on today's psy complex. Throughout the ages, large bodies of medical and scientific literature have been devoted to medicalizing and pathologizing various behaviours, experiences, and physical characteristics as being indicative of deficiency, biological inferiority, and mental/physical illness. A Mad lens can help us see that once various groups are brought into being and constituted as types of Mad or disabled people (i.e. as 'inverts,' 'imbeciles,' 'idiots,' etc.) they are thereby dehumanized and subjected to exploitation such as "slavery, imprisonment, institutionalization, and state violence" (Clare, 2019, p. 4). This violence is in turn characterized as being necessary, correctional, curative, and/or therapeutic. Applying a Mad lens thereby shows us the ways in which sanism and ableism are mutually constitutive of white supremacy, cisheteropatriarchy, and other forms of oppression.

This chapter has outlined some possible responses to the question of what Mad Studies can help us understand. In the next chapter, I explore what Mad Studies can help us do. As will be seen, Mad Studies is, at its core, action oriented. The purpose of Mad Studies is not just to understand things differently, but to provide some of the tools for taking action and making change within the systems that create marginalization.

ACKNOWLEDGEMENTS

Sections of this chapter draw on two chapters, listed below, from Pilling, M. D. (2022*) Queer and trans madness: Struggles for social justice*. Palgrave Macmillan. Reproduced with permission of Palgrave Springer Nature.

Introduction: Queer and trans madness: Struggles for social justice

Expanding the struggle against queer and trans pathologization: Challenging biomedicalism

---

Recommended resources

Abdillahi, I., Meerai, S., & Poole, J. (2017). When the suffering is compounded: Towards anti-Black sanism. In S. Wehbi & H. Parada (Eds.), *Reimagining anti-oppression social work practice* (pp. 109–122). Canadian Scholars Press.

Clare, E. (2019). Defective and deficient: White supremacy and disability oppression tangled together. *Understanding and dismantling privilege*, 9(1), 1–7.

LeBlanc, S., & Kinsella, E. A. (2016). Toward epistemic justice: A critically reflexive examination of 'sanism' and implications for knowledge generation. *Studies in Social Justice, 10*(1), 59–78. https://doi.org/10.26522/ssj.v10i1.1324

Yellow Bird, P. (2004). *Wild Indians: Native perspectives on the Hiawatha Asylum for Insane Indians.* National Empowerment Center. https://power2u.org/wp-content/uploads/2017/01/NativePerspectives-PeminaYellowBird.pdf

NOTES

1 In other words, if we were to employ this binary way of thinking, the many different ways that various Mad activists and scholars take up madness could be seen as falling between these two extremes. For example, the social model of disability (which is sometimes applied to madness) could be said to fall somewhere within the shades of gray given that some iterations of it include conceptualizations of 'impairment' as biological and 'disability' as socially produced, a distinction that has been critiqued by some Mad scholars for reinforcing biological essentialism and the medicalization of madness (Beresford & Wallcraft, 1997; Nabbali, 2009).

2 This idea is inspired by the gender galaxy model (see https://translanguageprimer.com/gender-galaxy/).

3 Johnk (2021) explains that an earlier conceptualization of bodymindspirit can be found in the work of Gloria Anzaldua and uses this as an example of Mad Studies' origins in women of colour feminisms.

4 The mainstream use of 'stigma' should be seen as distinct from sociological theorizing of the concept, such as Goffman's (1963).

REFERENCES

Abdillahi, I., Meerai, S., & Poole, J. (2017). When the suffering is compounded: Towards anti-Black sanism. In S. Wehbi & H. Parada (Eds.), *Reimagining anti-oppression social work practice* (pp. 109–122). Canadian Scholars Press.

Beresford, P. (2005). Social approaches to madness and distress: User perspectives and user knowledges. In J. Tew (Ed.), *Social perspectives in mental health: Developing social models to understand and work with mental distress* (pp. 32–52). Jessica Kingsley Publishers.

Beresford, P. (2020). 'Mad', Mad studies and advancing inclusive resistance. *Disability & Society, 35*(8), 1337–1342. https://doi.org/10.1080/09687599.2019.1692168

Beresford, P. & Rose, D. (2023). Decolonising global mental health: The role of Mad Studies. *Cambridge Prisms: Global Mental Health, 10,* e30. https://doi.org/10.1017/gmh.2023.21

Beresford, P., & Wallcraft, J. (1997). Psychiatric system survivors and emancipatory research: Issues, overlaps and differences. In C. Barnes & G. Mercer, *Doing disability research* (pp. 66–87). The Disability Press.

Birnbaum, M. (1960). The right to treatment. *American Bar Association Journal, 46*(5), 499–505.

Boyle, M. (2011). Making the world go away, and how psychology and psychiatry benefit. In M. Rapley, J. Moncrieff, & J. Dillon (Eds.), *De-medicalizing misery: Psychiatry, psychology and the human condition* (pp. 27–44). Palgrave Macmillan. https://doi.org/10.1057/9780230342507

Bruce, L. M. J. (2021). *How to go mad without losing your mind: madness and black radical creativity.* Duke University Press. https://doi.org/10.2307/j.ctv1ks0hp4

Burstow, B. (2015). *Psychiatry and the business of madness: An ethical and epistemological accounting.* Palgrave Macmillan. https://doi.org/10.1057/9781137503855

Butler, J. (2004). *Undoing gender.* Routledge. https://doi.org/10.4324/9780203499627

Costa, L. (2014, October 15). *Mad Studies – What it is and why you should care.* Mad Studies Network. https://mad-studies2014.wordpress.com/2014/10/15/mad-studies-what-it-is-and-why-you-should-care-2/

Chrisjohn, R. D., McKay, S. M., & Smith, A. O. (2017). *Dying to please you: Indigenous suicide in contemporary Canada.* Theytus Books Limited.

Clare, E. (2019). Defective and deficient: White supremacy and disability oppression tangled together. *Understanding and dismantling privilege, 9*(1), 1–7.

Cosantino, J. & Pilling, M. (2024, September 7). *Forging a MadTrans Studies* [Conference presentation]. The 2nd International Trans Studies Conference, Northwestern University, Evanston, IL, United States.

Cuthand, T. J. (n.d.). *Spotlight on Madness by Thirza Cuthand.* Akimbo. https://akimbo.ca/akimblog/spotlight-on-madness-by-thirza-cuthand/

Daley, A. (2021). Narrating genders in psychiatric inpatient chart documentation. In A. Daley & M. D. Pilling (Eds.), *Interrogating psychiatric narratives of madness: Documented lives* (pp. 57–86). Palgrave MacMillan. https://doi.org/10.1007/978-3-030-83692-4_3

Deerinwater, J., Ho, S., Thompson, V., Wong, A., Erevelles, N., & Morrow, M. (2023). A conversation on disability justice and intersectionality. In M. H. Rioux, A. Buettgen, E. Zubrow, & J. Viera (Eds.), *Handbook of disability: Critical thought and social change in a globalizing world* (pp. 1–22). Springer. https://doi.org/10.1007/978-981-16-1278-7_95-1

Diamond, S. (2013). What makes us a community? Reflections on building solidarity in anti-sanist praxis. In B. A. LeFrançois, R. Menzies, & G. Reaume (Eds.), *Mad matters: A critical reader in Canadian Mad Studies* (pp. 64–78). Canadian Scholars Press.

Diesfeld, K. & Sjöström, S. (2007). Interpretive flexibility: why doesn't insight incite controversy in mental health law? *Behavioral Sciences & the Law, 25*(1), 85–101. https://doi.org/10.1002/bsl.705

Doharty, N. (2024). Can Black Critical Theory sit with Mad Studies in Education in Britain? *Pedagogy, Culture & Society.* https://doi.org/10.1080/14681366.2024.2366287

Dwornik, A. (2021). The interface of Mad Studies and Indigenous ways of knowing: Innovation, co-creation, and decolonization. *Critical Social Work, 22*(2), 24–39. https://doi.org/10.22329/csw.v22i2.7097

Eromosele, F. (2022). Madness, decolonialization and mental health activism in Africa. In P. Beresford and J. Russo (Eds.), *The*

Routledge international handbook of Mad Studies (pp. 327–339). Routledge. https://doi.org/10.4324/9780429465444-38

Ezell, J. (2019). "Returning forest darlings": Gay liberationist sanctuary in the Southeastern network, 1973–80. *Radical History Review, 2019*(135), 71–94. https://doi.org/10.1215/01636545-7607833

Fausto-Sterling, A. (2000). *Sexing the body: Gender politics and the construction of sexuality*. Basic Books.

Fernando, S. (2010). *Mental health, race and culture*. Palgrave Macmillan. https://doi.org/10.1007/978-1-137-01368-2

Fernando, S. (2017). *Institutional racism in psychiatry and clinical psychology*. Palgrave Macmillan. https://doi.org/10.1007/978-3-319-62728-1

Fricker, M. (2007). *Epistemic injustice: Power and the ethics of knowing*. Oxford University Press. https://doi.org/10.1093/acprof:oso/9780198237907.001.0001

Fricker, M. (2010). Replies to Alcoff, Goldberg, and Hookway on Epistemic Injustice. *Episteme, 7*(2), 164–178. https://doi.org/10.3366/epi.2010.0006

Galasiński, D. & Ziółkowska, J. (2013). Managing information: Misrepresentation in the patient's notes. *Qualitative Inquiry, 19*(8), 589–599. https://doi.org/10.1177/1077800413494346

Gender galaxy. (n.d.). The Trans Language Primer. https://translanguageprimer.com/gender-galaxy/

Gilman, S. L. (1985). *Difference and pathology: Stereotypes of sexuality, race, and madness*. Cornell University Press.

Goffman, E. (1963). *Stigma: Notes on the management of spoiled identity*. Prentice-Hall.

Gorman, R. (2013). Thinking through race, class, and mad identity politics. In B. A. LeFrançois, R. Menzies, & G. Reaume (Eds.), *Mad matters: A critical reader in Canadian Mad Studies* (pp. 269–280). Canadian Scholars Press.

Gorman, R. & LeFrançois, B. A. (2017). Mad Studies. In B. M. Z. Cohen (Ed.), *Routledge international handbook of critical mental health* (pp. 107–114). Routledge. https://doi.org/10.4324/9781315399584-14

Gorman, R., saini, a., Tam, L., Udegbe, O., & Usar, O. (2013). Mad people of colour: A manifesto. *Asylum: An International Magazine for Democratic Psychiatry, 20*(4), 27. https://asylummagazine.org/2013/12/mad-people-of-color-a-manifesto-by-rachel-gorman-annu-saini-louise-tam-onyin yechukwu-udegbe-onar-usar/

Hamilton, B. & Roper, C. (2006). Troubling 'insight': power and possibilities in mental health care. *Journal of Psychiatric and Mental Health Nursing, 13*(4), 416–422. https://doi.org/10.1111/j.1365-2850.2006.00997.x

Harper, V. (1988). Them crazy Indians. In B. Burstow & D. Weitz (Eds.), *Shrink resistant: The struggle against psychiatry in Canada* (pp. 121–125). New Star Books.

Høyer, G. (2000). On the justification for civil commitment. *Acta Psychiatrica Scandinavica, 101*(399), 65–71. https://doi.org/10.1111/j.0902-4441.2000.007s020[dash]16.x

Howell, A. (2018). Forget "militarization": Race, disability and the "martial politics" of the police and of the university. *International Feminist Journal of Politics, 20*(2), 117–136. https://doi.org/10.1080/14616742.2018.1447310

Jackson, V. (2002). In our own voice: African-American stories of oppression, survival and recovery in mental health systems. *International Journal of Narrative Therapy and Community Work, 2*, 11–31.

Johnk, L. (2021). *Shifting roots: Reimagining the genealogical roots of Disability Studies and Mad Studies through women of color feminisms* [Doctoral dissertation, Oregon State University]. Scholars Archive.

Joseph, A. J. (2014). A prescription for violence: The legacy of colonization in contemporary forensic mental health and the production of difference. *Critical Criminology, 22*(2), 273–292. https://doi.org/10.1007/s10612-013-9208-1

Joseph, A. J. (2015). The necessity of an attention to Eurocentrism and colonial technologies: An addition to critical mental health literature. *Disability & Society, 30*(7), 1021–1041. https://doi.org/10.1080/09687599.2015.1067187

Joseph, A. J. (2019). Constituting "lived experience" discourses in mental health: The ethics of racialized identification/

representation and the erasure of intergeneration colonial violence. *Journal of Ethics in Mental Health, 10,* 1–23.

Kanani, N. (2011). Race and madness: Locating the experiences of racialized people with psychiatric histories in Canada and the United States. *Critical Disability Discourse, 3,* 1–14.

Knight, S., Jarvis, G. E., Ryder, A. G., Lashley, M., & Rousseau, C. (2022). Ethnoracial differences in coercive referral and intervention among patients with first-episode psychosis. *Psychiatric Services, 73*(1), 2–8. https://doi.org/10.1176/appi.ps.202000715

Lavallée, K. (2022, August 30). *Spirit injury and the healing journey* [Video]. Major Research Paper Dissemination, Toronto Metropolitan University. YouTube. https://youtu.be/m15Ivbn9_aM?si=QQkdtAIylhz3Mf0u

Lavallée, L. (2021, January 12). *Spirit injuries: Indigenous perspectives of mental health* [Video]. Network Environments for Indigenous Health Research Ontario Webinar, Waakebiness-Bryce Institute for Indigenous Health, Dalla Lana School of Public Health, University of Toronto. YouTube. https://youtu.be/Jul3glN3UH4?si=tCyPM_y0wueRLJd0

Lavallée, L. F. & Poole, J. M. (2010). Beyond recovery: Colonization, health and healing for Indigenous people in Canada. *International Journal of Mental Health and Addiction, 8,* 271–281.

LeBlanc, S. & Kinsella, E. A. (2016). Toward epistemic justice: A critically reflexive examination of 'sanism' and implications for knowledge generation. *Studies in Social Justice, 10*(1), 59–78. https://doi.org/10.26522/ssj.v10i1.1324

LeFrançois, B. A., Menzies, R., & Reaume, G. (Eds.). (2013). *Mad matters: A critical reader in Canadian Mad Studies.* Canadian Scholars Press.

LeFrançois, B. A., Beresford, P., & Russo, J. (2016). Destination Mad Studies. *Intersectionalities: A Global Journal of Social Work Analysis, Research, Polity, and Practice, 5*(3), 1–10. https://journals.library.mun.ca/ojs/index.php/IJ/article/view/1690/1342

LeFrançois, B. A., & Voronka, J. (2022). Mad epistemologies and maddening the ethics of knowledge production. In T.

Macías (Ed.), *Unravelling research: The ethics and politics of research in the social sciences* (pp. 105–130). Fernwood Publishing.

Lewis, B. (2006). *Moving beyond Prozac, DSM, and the new psychiatry: The birth of postpsychiatry.* University of Michigan Press. https://doi.org/10.3998/mpub.93209

Liegghio, M. (2013). A denial of being: Psychiatrization as epistemic violence. In B. A. LeFrançois, R. Menzies, & G. Reaume (Eds.), *Mad matters: A critical reader in Canadian Mad Studies* (pp. 122–129). Canadian Scholars Press.

Linklater, R. (2014). *Decolonizing trauma work: Indigenous stories and strategies.* Fernwood Publishing.

Mannoe, M. (2023). Confronting ableism and sanism in policing: An interview with Vesper Moore. *Pivot Legal Society.* www.pivotlegal.org/confronting_ableism_sanism_in_policing

Meerai, S., Abdillahi, I., & Poole, J. (2016). An introduction to anti-Black sanism. *Intersectionalities: A Global Journal of Social Work Analysis, Research, Polity, and Practice, 5*(3), 18–35. https://doi.org/10.32920/21751496

Menzies, R. & Palys, T. (2006). Turbulent spirits: Aboriginal patients in the British Columbia psychiatric system, 1879–1950. In J. Moran & D. Wright (Eds.), *Mental health and Canadian society: Historical perspectives* (pp. 149–175). McGill-Queen's University Press. https://doi.org/10.1515/9780773576544-010

Menzies, R., LeFrançois, B. A., & Reaume, G. (2013). Introducing Mad Studies. In B. A. LeFrançois, R. Menzies, & G. Reaume, *Mad matters: A critical reader in Canadian Mad Studies* (pp. 1–26). Canadian Scholars Press.

Metzl, J. M. (2009). *The protest psychosis: How schizophrenia became a Black disease.* Beacon Press.

Metzl, J. M., McClelland, S. I., & Bergner, E. (2016). Conflations of marital status and sanity: Implicit heterosexist bias in psychiatric diagnosis in physician-dictated charts at a Midwestern medical center. *The Yale Journal of Biology and Medicine, 89*(2), 247–254.

Mills, C. (2014). *Decolonizing global mental health: The psychiatrization of the majority world*. Routledge. https://doi.org/10.4324/9780203796757

Morrow, M. (2013). Recovery: Progressive paradigm or neoliberal smokescreen? In B. A. LeFrançois, R. Menzies, & G. Reaume (Eds.), *Mad matters: A critical reader in Canadian Mad Studies* (pp. 323–333). Canadian Scholars Press.

Mosby, I. (2013). Administering colonial science: Nutrition research and human biomedical experimentation in Aboriginal communities and residential schools, 1942–1952. *Histoire sociale/Social history*, 46(1), 145–172. https://doi.org/10.1353/his.2013.0015

Nabbali, E. M. (2009). A "mad" critique of the social model of disability. *International Journal of Diversity in Organizations, Communities, and Nations*, 9(4), 1. https://doi.org/10.18848/1447-9532/cgp/v09i04/39702

Nasser, S. (2020a, June 1). Security footage retrieved from highrise where Toronto woman fell to her death. *CBC News*. www.cbc.ca/news/canada/toronto/regis-korchinski-paquet-toronto-1.5593718

Nasser, S. (2020b, November 3). Members of LGBTQ community demand answers after Black trans woman dies in police custody. *CBC News*. https://cbc.ca/news/canada/toronto/black-trans-woman-crisis-toronto-siu-1.5787990

Nasser, S. (2023, July 10). Police in Ontario killed a man in crisis. Now they're fighting to keep their names private. *CBCNews*. https://cbc.ca/news/canada/toronto/ejaz-choudry-lawsuit-police-names-1.6898010

Nelson, S. (2012). *Challenging hidden assumptions: Colonial norms as determinants of Aboriginal mental health*. National Collaborating Centre for Aboriginal Health. https://ccnsa-nccah.ca/docs/determinants/FS-ColonialNorms-Nelson-EN.pdf

Ojanuga, D. (1993). The medical ethics of the 'father of gynaecology', Dr J Marion Sims. *Journal of Medical Ethics*, 19(1), 28–31. https://doi.org/10.1136/jme.19.1.28

Pattadath, B. (2016). Experience as 'expert' knowledge: A critical understanding of survivor research in mental health. *Philosophy, Psychiatry, & Psychology, 23*(3), 203–205. https://doi.org/10.1353/ppp.2016.0018

Perlin, M. L. (1992). On sanism. *SMU Law Review, 46*, 373–407.

Persaud, S. (2022). *No sovereign remedy: Distress, madness, and mental health care in Guyana* [Doctoral dissertation, York University]. YorkSpace.

Pilling, M. D., Daley, A., Gibson, M. F., Ross, L. E., & Zaheer, J. (2018). Assessing "insight," determining agency and autonomy: Implicating social identities. In J. M. Kilty & E. Dej (Eds.), *Containing madness: Gender and "psy" in institutional contexts* (pp. 191–213). Palgrave Macmillan. https://doi.org/10.1007/978-3-319-89749-3_9

Pilling, M. D. (2021). Sexual violence and psychosis: Intersections of rape culture, sanism, and anti-Black sanism in psychiatric inpatient chart documentation. In A. Daley & M. D. Pilling (Eds.), *Interrogating psychiatric narratives of madness: Documented lives* (pp. 137–164). Palgrave Macmillan. https://doi.org/10.1080/02650533.2023.2207728

Pilling, M. D. (2022). *Queer and trans madness: Struggles for social justice*. Palgrave MacMillan. https://doi.org/10.1007/978-3-030-90413-5

Pilling, M. D. (Forthcoming). Toward mad trans liberation: The necessity of a mad-queer-trans lens. In B. A. LeFrançois, I. Abdillahi, G. Reaume, & R. Menzies (Eds.). *Mad Matters: A Critical Reader in Canadian Mad Studies (Second Edition)*. Canadian Scholars Press.

Poole, J., Jivraj, T., Arslanian, A., Bellows, K., Chiasson, S., Hakimy, H., Passini, J. & Reid, J. (2012) Sanism, "mental health", and social work/education: A review and call to action. *Intersectionalities: A Global Journal of Social Work Analysis, Research, Polity, and Practice, 1*(1), 20–36. https://doi.org/10.32920/21751490.v1

Porter, R. (2002). *Madness: A brief history*. Oxford University Press.

Price, M. (2011). *Mad at school: Rhetorics of mental disability and academic life*. University of Michigan Press. https://doi.org/10.3998/mpub.1612837

Price, M. (2015). The bodymind problem and the possibilities of pain. *Hypatia, 30*(1), 268–284. https://doi.org/10.1111/hypa.12127

Rapley, M., Moncrieff, J., & Dillon, J. (2011). Carving nature at its joints? DSM and the medicalization of everyday life. In M. Rapley, J. Moncrieff, & J. Dillon (Eds.), *De-medicalizing misery: Psychiatry, psychology and the human condition* (pp. 1–10). Palgrave Macmillan. https://doi.org/10.1057/9780230342507_1

Reaume, G. (2002). Lunatic to patient to person: Nomenclature in psychiatric history and the influence of patients' activism in North America. *International Journal of Law and Psychiatry, 25*(4), 405–426. https://doi.org/10.1016/S0160-2527(02)00130-9

Reaume, G. (2022). How is Mad Studies different from antipsychiatry and critical psychiatry? In P. Beresford and J. Russo (Eds.), *The Routledge international handbook of Mad Studies* (pp. 98–107). Routledge. https://doi.org/10.4324/9780429465444-15

Rimke, H. (2016). Introduction – Mental and emotional distress as a social justice issue: Beyond psychocentrism. *Studies in Social Justice, 10*(1), 4–17. https://doi.org/10.26522/ssj.v10i1.1407

Rimke, H. (2018). Sickening institutions: A feminist sociological analysis and critique of religion, medicine, and psychiatry. In J. M. Kilty & E. Dej (Eds.), *Containing madness: Gender and 'psy' in institutional contexts* (pp. 15–39). Palgrave Macmillan. https://doi.org/10.1007/978-3-319-89749-3_2

Rimke, H. & Hunt, A. (2002). From sinners to degenerates: The medicalization of morality in the 19th century. *History of the Human Sciences, 15*(1), 59–88. https://doi.org/10.1177/0952695102015001073

Ringer, A. & Holen, M. (2016). "Hell no, they'll think you're mad as a hatter": Illness discourses and their implications for patients in mental health practice. *Health, 20*(2), 161–175. https://doi.org/10.1177/1363459315574115

Russo, J. (2023). Psychiatrization, assertions of epistemic justice, and the question of agency. *Frontiers in Sociology, 8*(1092298). https://doi.org/10.3389/fsoc.2023.1092298

Schalk, S. (2018). *Bodyminds reimagined:(Dis)ability, race, and gender in Black women's speculative fiction*. Duke University Press. https://doi.org/10.1215/9780822371830

Schalk, S. (2022). *Black disability politics*. Duke University Press. https://doi.org/10.1215/9781478027003

Somerville, S. (2000). *Queering the color line: Race and the invention of homosexuality in American culture*. Duke University Press. https://doi.org/10.1215/9780822378761

Sharma, P. (2022). Navigating voices, politics, positions amidst peers: Resonances and dissonances in India. In P. Beresford and J. Russo (Eds.), *The Routledge international handbook of Mad Studies* (pp. 340–350). Routledge. https://doi.org/10.4324/9780429465444-39

Spandler, H. (2017). Mad and Queer Studies, shared visions? *Asylum: An International Magazine for Democratic Psychiatry, 24*(1), 5–6.

Spandler, H. & Barker, M. J. (2016, July 1). *Mad and Queer Studies: Interconnections and tensions*. Mad Studies Network. https://madstudies2014.wordpress.com/2016/07/01/mad-and-queer-studies-interconnections-and-tensions/

Spandler, H. & Poursanidou, D. (2019). Who is included in the Mad Studies project? *The Journal of Ethics in Mental Health, 10*.

Timimi, S. (2011). Globalising mental health: a neo-liberal project. *Ethnicity and Inequalities in Health and Social Care, 4*(3), 155–160. https://doi.org/10.1108/17570981111249293

Tosh, J. (2017). Gender non-conformity or psychiatric non-compliance? How organized non-compliance can offer a future without psychiatry. In M. Morrow & L. H. Malcoe (Eds.), *Critical inquiries for social justice in mental health* (pp. 255–282). University of Toronto Press. https://doi.org/10.3138/9781442619708-011

Voronka, J. (2016). The politics of 'people with lived experience': Experiential authority and the risks of strategic essentialism. *Philosophy, Psychiatry, & Psychology, 23*(3), 189–201. https://doi.org/10.1353/ppp.2016.0017

Waldram, J. B. (2004). *Revenge of the Windigo; The construction of the mind and mental health of North American Aboriginal peoples.* University of Toronto Press. https://doi.org/10.3138/9781442683815

Waldron, I. R. G. (2021). The wounds that do not heal: Black expendability and the traumatizing aftereffects of anti-Black police violence. *Equality, Diversity and Inclusion, 40*(1), 29–40. https://doi.org/10.1108/EDI-06-2020-0175

Walker, D. E. (2022). *Coyote's Swing: A memoir and critique of mental hygiene in Native America.* Washington State University Press.

Washington, H. A. (2006). *Medical apartheid: The dark history of medical experimentation on Black Americans from colonial times to the present.* Doubleday Books.

Whitaker, R. (2001). *Mad in America: Bad science, bad medicine, and the enduring mistreatment of the mentally ill.* Basic Books. https://doi.org/10.1176/appi.ps.54.1.112

Yellow Bird, P. (2004). *Wild Indians: Native perspectives on the Hiawatha Asylum for Insane Indians.* National Empowerment Center. https://power2u.org/wp-content/uploads/2017/01/NativePerspectivesPeminaYellowBird.pdf

WHAT CAN MAD STUDIES HELP US DO?

This chapter asks what Mad Studies can help us do and explores various aspects of Mad Studies as forms of praxis. Praxis is where theory and action meet; when we engage in praxis, we combine reflection and action to enact social change and work towards collective liberation (Freire, 1972). Costa and Ross (2023) argue that Mad Studies "is itself praxis" because Mad theory aims to articulate, mobilize, and realize the emancipatory objectives of the Mad movement (p. 4). Originating as it does in community activism, Mad Studies is action-oriented and can provide tools for doing things differently. Therefore, following Costa and Ross (2023), the premise of this chapter is that Mad Studies is praxis. The chapter begins with an exploration of the praxis-oriented aspects of employing a Mad lens, including the use of madness as an analytic, and the creation of survivor research. The rest of the chapter focuses on various other aspects of Mad praxis, including a section on Mad pedagogy, and another on Mad art as praxis. The final section covers how Mad people resist psychiatric violence, including through creating different approaches to care and treatment. This includes a discussion of resistance to coercive care and electroconvulsive therapy (ECT), and an exploration of the Mad practice of peer support and its struggles with co-option.

DOI: 10.4324/9781003561552-4

EMPLOYING A MAD LENS AS PRAXIS

At the end of Chapter 2 I explained what a Mad lens helps us understand, arguing that it can be employed to illuminate existing knowledge about madness and Mad people in a different light. Mad people have been subject to scrutiny, objectification, dehumanization, and violence in the name of knowledge production. This violence is rarely recognized as such and has been characterized as neutral and objective, and often as necessary and beneficial. Chapter 2 shows how using a Mad lens to examine such knowledge exposes its violent underpinnings and demonstrates how it serves the interests of white supremacy and cisheteropatriarchy. The following will expand on this understanding of a Mad lens and explore its praxis-oriented aspects; that is, what a Mad lens helps us do. I explain some of the ways in which a Mad lens can be used as a way of knowing, and as a means of creating knowledge that facilitates Mad ways of doing and resisting. However, it should be noted that what a Mad lens helps us understand and what it helps us do are very much intertwined and cannot be fully teased apart.

Focusing on the praxis-oriented aspects of using a Mad lens shows that when a Mad lens is employed, Mad people are no longer specimens to be examined by supposedly dispassionate outsiders. Rather, Mad knowledge is positioned as valuable expertise, and as ways of seeing and knowing that can do a number of things, including exposing the violence of the biomedical model and resisting the dominance of the psy complex. As Spandler and Poursanidou (2019) put it, a Mad lens "does not treat madness as an 'object of study' (i.e. studying madness or Mad people) but rather as a potentially credible source of knowledge in its own right" (p. 11). As they go on to explain, a Mad lens mobilizes "Mad knowledge and subjectivity as a tool of understanding and analysis – an instrument of knowing," which is important because Mad knowledge has rarely been seen "as credible … *on its own terms*" (Spandler & Poursanidou, 2019, p. 11, emphasis in original). As will be discussed, this reclamation of Mad knowledge can be seen as a form of epistemic justice.

MADNESS AS AN ANALYTIC: MADDENING EPISTEMOLOGIES

Madness can be employed as an analytic, that is, to 'madden.' 'Maddening' can be thought of as being analogous to, and intersecting with, 'cripping' or 'queering,' though each have their own specific genealogies, meanings, and uses (Kafer, 2013; Price, 2015; Thorneycroft, 2020; McRuer, 2006). To madden is to use madness as an epistemology. In other words, to madden is to employ the logic, or perhaps the anti-logic, of Mad Studies and Mad knowledge to any given topic or query. This does not require self-identification as Mad. Just as anyone might engage in 'queering' or 'cripping,' so might any person engage in 'maddening.' Maddening must be seen as a form of praxis because it is a way of fighting back and resisting the objectification and dehumanization imposed by conventional scholarship on mental health and illness. As LeFrançois and Voronka (2022) put it, "Mad Studies, at its most maddening and unruly, serves to resist normalcy and disrupt the dominant sanist and racist definitions of madness typically used in 'mental illness' research whilst calling in to question enlightenment notions of rationality" (p. 106). Importantly, the practice of maddening is not a one-way directional analysis. Maddening often involves a more complex and reciprocal relationship. To madden is to be unruly, to flaunt disciplinary boundaries, to co-mingle with other critical ways of knowing, allowing each to change the other and become something new.

The use of 'maddening' as an analytic is still "under-explored and under-theorised" (Thorneycroft, 2020), however, it is on the rise. For example, Doharty (2024) argues for a maddening of Black Critical Theory in the context of creating knowledge about the experiences of Black students in Britain. Maddening Black Critical Theory can illuminate the ways in which Black students are placed outside of 'the human' and Reason, as well as how anti-Blackness creates distress and invalidates Mad Black knowledge (Doharty, 2024). A maddened Black Critical Theory challenges the predominant discourses perpetuated by mental health literature that "decontextualizes and pathologises Black suffering" and instead acknowledges and seeks to abolish the conditions that create distress for Black students (Doharty, 2024, p. 1).

Other examples of the use of maddening include efforts to madden the fields of Black speculative fiction (Pickens, 2019), Early Childhood Education (Davies, 2022, 2023), Fat Studies (Shanouda, 2023), Game Studies (Rodéhn, 2022), Literary Studies (McEwen, 2022; Wolframe, 2014), as well as calls to madden the academy more broadly (Cea-Madrid & Castillo-Parada, 2021; Krazinski et al., 2023). There are also implicit uses of madness as a way of knowing. I discuss elsewhere how the use of a mad-queer-trans lens can be used to create different ways of knowing than those perpetuated by conventional lesbian, gay, bisexual, trans, and queer (LGBTQ) mental health research (Pilling, 2022). This can be seen as a form of 'maddening' knowledge about queer and trans experiences of distress. So far, the practice of maddening has mostly been focused on issues pertaining to the psy complex. However, the use of madness as an analytic does not necessarily need to be restricted to such topics and will perhaps become broader in scope over time.

SURVIVOR RESEARCH: RECLAIMING EXPERTISE AND WORKING TOWARDS EPISTEMIC JUSTICE

Survivor research can be seen as another praxis-oriented use of a Mad lens. Survivor research predates Mad Studies and is a field of study in its own right, however, the two are entwined (Sweeney, 2016). Like Mad Studies, survivor research in Canada arose from the Mad movement. Landry (2017) dates the first instances of documented survivor research in Canada to the 1990s and explains that Canadian survivor research emerged from the Mad movement but has also been influenced by survivor research created in the United Kingdom (UK), where it is more prevalent (p. 1439). Mad Studies and survivor research are both critical of the psy complex and demonstrate how madness and distress are caused by "the social conditions of poverty, oppression, systemic violence, trauma, and a *lack* of adequate, accessible supports and resources"

(Landry, 2017, p. 1452, emphasis in original). This differs from mainstream mental health research, much of which is medical in nature and perpetuates the biomedical model (Beresford & Wallcraft, 1997; Beresford & Rose, 2009). Like Mad Studies, survivor research is driven by the desire to make a difference to the material conditions that create inequity for those deemed Mad. It centres the perspectives, needs, and experiences of service users, thereby shifting research priorities and goals to reflect an "emancipatory paradigm" that foregrounds social change as the main objective of conducting research (Landry, 2017, p. 1447).

Survivor research is also sometimes referred to as 'service user research,' or more simply as 'user research.' These terms are employed differently by different people and should be defined at the outset by research teams employing these terms (Faulkner, 2004, p. 4). Some position the term 'user research' as a specific term that refers to research conducted by and for those who have used mental health systems, and 'survivor research' as a broader term that includes Mad people who may or may not have lived experienced of mental health services (Faulkner, 2004, p. 2). 'Survivor' (short for 'psychiatric survivor') also tends to be a more politicized term that can indicate a critical stance towards psychiatric services (i.e. one is a survivor of the oppressive psy complex).

A key aspect of survivor research is that it is controlled by those who have experienced distress and/or the mental health system. Survivors/service users play an essential role in all aspects of the research process, from inception to completion (Russo, 2012). This differs from mainstream mental health research that employs survivors/service users as research subjects or as advisors with little power over major decisions governing the research process (Ormerod et al., 2018; Ross et al., 2023; Ross & Pilling, 2024). Survivor research thereby challenges who is considered to have expertise and places power in the hands of survivors/service users instead of medical professionals. As explained in Chapter 2, Mad people have been positioned as lacking reason, as incapable of knowing reality or even their own experiences and bodymind; in other words, Mad people experience epistemic injustice. Survivor research can be seen as a pathway to epistemic justice because it positions Mad people as knowing subjects with valuable insights and the capacity to create social change. This counters the ways Mad people have been made knowable through ableist, racist, transphobic (and otherwise oppressive) medical discourses and diagnoses. Survivor research increases Mad people's credibility and status as 'legitimate knowers' through the creation of an evidence base that is conceived of, and controlled by, survivors rather than by medical professionals (Beresford & Rose, 2009).

SIMILARITIES TO FEMINIST RESEARCH

Survivor research has many similarities to feminist research (and, of course, some survivor research *is* feminist research). Like feminist research, it challenges the positivist paradigm underlying mainstream research. Survivor research belies the notion of 'objectivity' and posits that all research is subjective in that it is created by humans and therefore reflects social worldviews, values, and perspectives. Survivor research is reflexive, which means that researchers acknowledge their positionality and how it is connected to power relations within and outside of the research process (Faulkner, 2004). Instead of trying to maintain a false sense of neutrality and objective distance, survivor research posits that shared identity between researchers and those being researched can improve the experience of research participants and the quality of research outcomes (Faulkner, 2004; Rose, 2001). As this indicates, survivor research embraces the subjective nature of the research process, and values lived experience as an authoritative source of knowledge (Beresford & Rose, 2009; Faulkner, 2021; Russo, 2012). Furthermore, like feminist research, survivor research challenges what counts as evidence and the hierarchical valuing of the means of gathering evidence. Mainstream research operates on the assumption that there is a hierarchy of types of evidence, with randomized control trials (RCT) at the top. Survivor research shows that

RCTs are not always the best means of producing evidence about the experiences and priorities of service users/survivors. Survivor research often favours qualitative approaches for their ability to capture depth of meaning, while not discounting that quantitative approaches can be useful (Beresford & Rose, 2009; Jones et al., 2014; Landry, 2017; Rose, 2022).

LIMITATIONS OF SURVIVOR RESEARCH AND DANGERS OF CO-OPTION

Survivor research is not without pitfalls. Despite repeated observations about the lack of survivor research conducted by and for Indigenous, Black, and racialized communities and the necessity of centring such voices in future survivor research, this problem persists (Begum, 2006; Beresford & Rose, 2009; Blakey, 2005; Kalathil, 2009, 2013; Lovell-Norton et al., 2021; Rose, 2022; Sweeney, 2016; Trivedi, 2008; Turner & Beresford, 2005). Likewise, there is a dearth of queer and trans survivor-led projects (Carr, 2015). These exclusions are shortcomings of survivor research, given the high levels of pathologization and coerced treatment of Indigenous, Black, and racialized people (Kalathil, 2013) and the pathologization of trans and queer ways of being (Pilling, 2022, forthcoming). Survivor communities, and thereby survivor research, are not exempt from hierarchies and oppression such as anti-Black racism and transphobia (Kalathil, 2009, 2013; Lovell-Norton et al., 2021; Rose & Kalathil, 2019). Additionally, as explained in more detail in Chapter 2, a Mad (and survivor) identity does not appeal to all communities in the same way, especially Indigenous, Black, racialized, and two-spirit, lesbian, gay, bisexual, trans, and queer, and intersex (2SLGBTQI) communities. Since survivor research is tightly tied to survivor identity, it may be limited as a research framework for communities who do not relate to this identity. White-centricity and hetero/cisnormativity within survivor research must be interrogated and challenged. Likewise, the construction of survivor as an identity does not have the same currency in some Global South contexts, raising questions about Eurocentricity and the transnational relevance of survivor research (Davar, 2015; Kalathil & Jones, 2016).

Survivor research is also limited by a lack of resources and funding. Survivor-led entities such as the Survivor Researcher Network in the UK are an integral part of maintaining a social justice lens and critical survivor voices in research rather than such voices becoming co-opted and subsumed by mainstream mental health research. However, such endeavours often run on volunteer labour and are under-resourced. Due to a lack of resources, survivor research often needs to find a home in non-survivor-led organizations or in academia. However, the goals, values, ethics, and methods of survivor research conflict with dominant academic culture and can easily be deemed too radical or unscientific (Beresford & Rose, 2009; Rose, 2023; Sweeney, 2016; Voronka & King, 2023). Likewise, neoliberal values in the academy result in the dominance of conservative perspectives in mental health research (Cohen, 2016; Lovell-Norton et al., 2021).

There are increasing demands from funders to include survivor (or 'patient') voices in research, and in the UK, this is mandated (Rose & Beresford, 2024). However, funders often favour co-production models that place much of the decision-making power in the hands of non-survivor lead investigators. Co-production models that do not employ Mad Studies are especially susceptible to ignoring ongoing legacies of harm perpetuated by the psy complex (Carr, 2022; Russo, 2023; Ross & Pilling, 2024). As such, the research inquiry at the heart of many projects that employ co-production revolves around service improvement rather than interrogating how such services can inflict harm (Sweeney, 2016). Co-production models such as patient and public involvement (PPI) in the UK and peer research in Canada are at risk of co-opting and subverting some of the central values of survivor research. For example, such models often (though not always) shift the locus of power to non-survivor lead investigators and espouse selective inclusion of survivor voices and priorities rather than centring them (Recovery in the Bin, 2018; Ormerod et al., 2018;

Papoulias & Callard, 2021; Rose et al., 2018; Ross et al., 2023). PPI and peer research often rely on contract labour, creating positions for survivors that are precarious and often exploitative (MacKinnon et al., 2021; Papoulias & Callard, 2022). While survivor research is closely tied to Mad Studies and its critique of the biomedical model, PPI and peer research do not necessarily always share these critiques (Ormerod et al., 2018). While some forms of PPI and peer research may accomplish emancipatory goals, others may claim to challenge the status quo through the performative inclusion of survivors while replicating the goals of the psy complex rather than challenging them (Ross & Pilling, 2024). It is crucial to support survivor-led research entities to prevent the co-option of critical survivor voices in research, and to maintain the emancipatory politics of survivor research that have the potential to disrupt business as usual in academia and the psy complex. Without adequate funding, the scope and impact of survivor research, and thereby Mad knowledge, is limited. Funding structures are one way in which Mad knowledge and the fight for epistemic justice can be curtailed and neutralized. Indeed, Mad knowledge, Mad Studies, and survivor research in academia and elsewhere are tenuous and vulnerable to co-option and elimination (Kalathil & Jones, 2016; Macintosh, 2023). This underscores the need for Mad praxis that maintains a strong critique of the psy complex and works towards emancipatory goals.

MAD PEDAGOGY

Mad pedagogy is another form of praxis that challenges epistemic injustice by reconfiguring who is seen as a legitimate knower, and questioning what counts as expertise. Mad pedagogy could be used anywhere, however, much of what has been written about it concerns Mad Studies courses delivered in university settings. Some exceptions include writing on early childhood education in Canada (Davies, 2022, 2023), and compulsory school level education in Britan (Doharty, 2024).

Mad Studies courses in universities are proliferating but are still relatively rare in comparison to the overwhelming majority of courses offered in the psy disciplines (and beyond) that employ the biomedical model to position madness as mental illness. University campuses are steeped in biomedical ideology and approaches to madness and distress. This is evident not only in the curriculum but in mental health wellness initiatives and university mental health strategies that mobilize individualizing approaches to mask structural and institutional violence (Kanani & Pilling, 2014; Landry & Church, 2016; Persaud et al., 2024). Mad students, Mad ways of knowing, and Mad emotions expressed on campus are positioned as risks in need of management (de Bie, 2019). Distressed students are pathologized and criminalized, as evidenced by the involvement of police and the routine use of handcuffs on distressed students (Neilson et al., 2019).

Mad Studies and Mad pedagogy can disrupt the biomedical monolith on campus and provide counter-narratives and critical interventions into sanism, ableism, and other interlocking oppressions. The importance of teaching and learning through an intersectional, anti-racist lens that explores the intersections of colonialism, anti-Black sanism (Abdillahi et al., 2017), and racism with ableism should be key to Mad pedagogy (Armstrong & Lefrançois, 2022; Poole & Grant, 2018; Reid & Poole, 2013; Roquemore & Cosantino, 2024). Mad pedagogy embraces uncertainty rather than mastery of any given subject area, exploring the messiness of difficult topics instead of packaging them neatly (Snyder et al. 2019; Castrodale, 2017). Below I outline some of the main considerations when it comes to Mad pedagogy including power and hierarchy in teaching and learning, Mad course design, accessibility and accommodations, and some of the limitations of Mad pedagogy.

POWER AND HIERARCHY IN TEACHING AND LEARNING

An essential element of Mad pedagogy is disrupting hierarchies and traditional power dynamics in teaching and learning. This involves challenging hierarchies of knowledge that discount Mad ways of knowing. This can be done by centring diverse Mad voices in the curriculum and through the presence of Mad activists and community members in the class as instructors, students, and/or guest speakers (Armstrong & LeFrançois, 2022; Church, 2013; Reville, 2013).

Mad pedagogy rejects the traditional role of instructor as all-knowing and students as passive learners lacking in expertise (Castrodale, 2017; Landry & Church, 2016; Roquemore & Cosantino, 2024). This may require some vulnerability on the part of the instructor in expressing and embracing uncertainty and refusing to self-position as the sole expert (Castrodale, 2017) or by engaging in pedagogical partnerships and co-creation practices with students (de Bie et al., 2019, 2022; Roquemore & Cosantino, 2024). For some Mad instructors, 'coming out' to students as Mad can be a powerful way to disrupt harmful assumptions about expertise and who is recognized as a legitimate knower (Landry & Church, 2016). However, the refusal to claim expertise and coming out as Mad is likely to be received differently from Indigenous, Black, racialized, queer, and trans instructors who face racism, queerphobia, and transphobia in their classrooms. While Mad pedagogy often involves taking risks, the level of risk for such instructors is higher, especially for those who are also untenured or precariously employed. Another means of diffusing instructor power is by remunerating activists, community leaders, and Indigenous elders to share knowledge with the class (Poole & Grant, 2018).

Mad pedagogy may increase some learners' self-knowledge and awareness of power relations. New or enhanced learning of structural sanism and other intersecting oppressions may provide opportunities to see life experiences and identity through a different (Mad) lens (Landry & Church, 2016). Some students gain insight into, and find new language to describe, the power of the psy complex over their lives. This may involve a paradigm shift in rejecting a deficit model and refusing to see themselves and others as burdensome, broken, or unworthy. Some may come out as Mad or as psychiatric survivors, while others may acquire an understanding of sanity and/or the avoidance of institutionalization as a form of privilege they had not previously considered (Castrodale, 2017; Reaume, 2006; Wolframe, 2012). This may lead to deepened knowledge of allyship, which can also be modelled by instructors (Church & Landry, 2017; Snyder et al., 2019).

Mad pedagogy positions learners as active, not only as knowledge producers in the classroom but as people who can effect social change (Ballantyne et al., 2020). This can lead students to examine their complicity in upholding and enforcing the carceral logic and practices of the psy complex (Snyder et al., 2019). This may be especially relevant to students in the 'helping professions' who may not have had an opportunity to challenge the "benign helper trope" (Snyder et al., 2019, p. 495). Mad pedagogy can illuminate how some practices that are constructed as help may in fact be harmful. Students can learn to centre survivors and work against harms, whether from within or outside the psy complex (Snyder et al., 2019).

MAD COURSE DESIGN

An important part of Mad pedagogy is in taking a different approach to course design. While there is no universal Mad approach, there are commonalities with course design informed by feminism, Disability Studies, trauma-informed frameworks, critical pedagogy, radical pedagogy, and anti-colonial approaches (Ballantyne et al., 2020; Burstow, 2003; Castrodale, 2017; Grant & Poole, 2018; Snyder et al., 2019). Mad pedagogues may employ elements of universal design, as well as innovative approaches from Disability Studies to create "pedagogical curb cuts" (Ben-Moshe et al., 2005). This may involve multiple ways of sharing information such as the use of various kinds of media (video, social media, blogs) and art (music, visual art, performance art) (Castrodale, 2019; Landry & Church, 2016; Newman et al., 2022; Reid et al., 2019; Reville, 2013). Taking a cue from Disability Studies, some employ arts-based means of learning and assessment such as photovoice, zine creation, and fine arts (Ballantyne et al., 2020; Carette et al., 2024; Mad Student Zine Team, 2022a, 2022b; Reid et al., 2019). Others employ a non-linear or "rhizomatic" course design to offer multiple entry points into course learning and move away from hierarchical course design (Snyder et al., 2019, p. 490). Mad pedagogy centres Mad knowledge and communities in various ways, such as featuring Mad narratives on the curriculum and through guest speakers (Armstrong & LeFrançois, 2022; Poole & Grant, 2018; Reaume, 2019; Reville, 2013). Some Mad pedagogues may do what they can to mitigate classism, prohibitive tuition fees, and credentialism by not placing pre-requisites on the course, offering scholarships and auditing opportunities to community members (Church, 2015; Reville, 2013, 2022), creating free courses for people with lived experience of the mental health system (Ballantyne et al., 2020) though there are significant barriers to doing so (Armstrong & Lefrançois, 2022).

ACCESSIBILITY AND ACCOMMODATIONS

Accommodation practices at universities assume that students are able-bodied unless they provide documented evidence of hegemonically legible forms of disability. Mad pedagogues can overturn this "sanist assumption" that students are non-disabled until proven otherwise by instead assuming that everyone is Mad and centring this assumption in course design and accommodation practices (Landry and Church, 2016, p. 180). Some strategies include flexibility with deadlines, avoiding morning time slots for classes, online modality, refusing to grade based on attendance, decreasing class sizes, and believing students' need for accommodations even if not made through official channels (Burstow, 2003; Poole & Grant, 2018; Roquemore & Cosantino, 2024; Snyder et al., 2019).

It is important to note that there are specific access considerations for learners with lived experience of mental health systems. Some such learners may be experiencing reactions to psychiatric drugs such as blurry vision, lethargy and fatigue, difficulty sitting still, and trouble with attention span, memory, and ability to concentrate (Burstow, 2003). Some Mad learners may hear voices, be engaged in "alternate realities," or become triggered or distressed in class. Those who have been institutionalized may also rightfully distrust authority (Burstow, 2003, p. 8). Some simple access strategies include using large font, building in frequent breaks, and ensuring one-on-one contact time (Burstow, 2003). However, expanding access for Mad students may require Mad pedagogues to learn and employ skills that many postsecondary instructors do not have and may not feel supported in using in a classroom context. These include visualization and grounding exercises, trigger management and de-escalation techniques, and introspection, amongst others (Burstow, 2003). It can also be helpful for instructors to have knowledge of the impact of trauma and how that may manifest, and how to validate seemingly unusual realities (Burstow, 2003).

LIMITATIONS OF MAD PEDAGOGY

There is much about academic life that is inimical to Mad people (de Bie, 2019; Price, 2011; Reville, 2013; Roquemore & Cosantino, 2024; Wolframe, 2012). Mad pedagogy in the university (and elsewhere) is constrained by the institution's norms, by-laws, and protocols (Church, 2015; Snyder et al., 2019). There are limitations on how far Mad pedagogues can stray from typical course design and accommodation practices. There are institutional barriers to implementing democratic principles and co-development design with Mad community members (Armstrong & Lefrançois, 2022). University instructors must navigate institutional demands and have various levels of power and support in doing so (Reville, 2013). For example, instructors are restricted by institutional grading deadlines, semester timelines, narrow accommodation practices, increasing class sizes and workloads, problematic ideas about what constitutes rigorous education, and the normalization and proliferation of punitive approaches to distressed students. Mad pedagogues consistently run up against common institutional ableist and sanist assumptions and practices. Even small adjustments that are commonly accepted among Disability Studies scholars (such as flexible deadlines and refusing attendance-based grading) may be difficult to implement in many university programs that have a limited understanding of accessibility.

Acquiring support for more radical accessibility practices that would truly make way for Mad learners and resist the criminalization of distressed students requires bigger shifts in institutional culture and priorities. This may lead some to conclude that Mad Studies and/or pedagogy is not possible in a university setting (Archibald, 2024). However, Mad pedagogy is a necessary (and precarious) intervention in higher education. Giving up on Mad pedagogy in the university allows the biomedical model to go relatively unchecked and primes students to perpetuate harm in the name of help. Mad pedagogy and pedagogues are also an important part of chipping away at pathologizing, criminalizing, and punitive approaches to Mad and distressed campus community members. Further resources and teaching tools for developing Mad educational content for postsecondary and upper-level secondary courses can be found on Madness Canada's Mad School website (https://madschool.ca/).

MAD CULTURAL PRODUCTION: MAD ART AS PRAXIS

Mad cultural production is a form of Mad praxis that is intricately tied to social movement organizing and creating social change (Kafai, 2021; Reid, 2018; Reid et al., 2019, Reid, 2019). Mad art can be a tool for mobilizing Mad knowledge and activism, and as such it can serve as a bridge between Mad academia and Mad communities (Reid et al., 2019). In Canada, Mad art has found a home in multidisciplinary disability arts non-profit organizations such as Tangled Art + Disability in Toronto, Ontario, and Kickstart Disability Arts and Culture in Vancouver British Columbia. Organizations such as Gallery Gachet in Vancouver, and Workman Arts in Toronto run art programs that centre mental health and support artists with lived experience of mental health and/or addiction services.

Mad art has largely been grounded within disability arts and culture, which uses disability "as a creative entry point" and forms new understandings of disability, deafhood, and madness (Chandler, 2019, p. 3). Disability arts is led by disabled, deaf, and Mad people and challenges deficit-based understandings of disability that are bound up with racist and colonial notions of defectiveness (Chandler, 2019; Kafai, 2021; Rice et al., 2021). Pathbreaking performance troupes such as Sins Invalid led by trans, disabled, and queer people of colour have reconfigured disability, madness, and deafhood outside of the biomedical model and reclaimed disabled queer of colour personhood as beautiful and essential (Kafai, 2021).

The connections between Mad art and disability arts are apparent, however, there may be advantages to exploring Mad art in its own right. Oftentimes, disability arts include Mad art as a minor focus. The full potential of Mad art as praxis has yet to be fully explored and disability arts does not adequately question, explicate, and challenge the links between Mad art and a biomedical framework (Reid et al., 2019). Mad artists draw attention to the history of the ways in which biomedical approaches have used art to surveil, diagnose, and pathologize Mad people (Reid et al., 2019; Walter, 2022). Reid et al. (2019) argue that, "early psy-based disciplines used creative production as a tool for diagnosing and charting deviant behaviours. It became a means for collecting information for assessment, creating opportunities for therapeutic (normalizing) outcomes, and as a documentation of client progress" (p. 258). Biomedical approaches have also framed art created by Mad people as a therapeutic tool rather than as necessitating skill and having merit and aesthetic value of its own (Reid, 2019; Walter, 2022).

Contemporary Mad artists reclaim Mad art from these biomedical roots. Indeed, Mad art can be a way to explore a more nuanced and complex view of madness and disrupt the biomedical gaze (Reid et al., 2019; Netchitailova, 2019). For example, Theo Jean Cuthand, a nêhiyaw (Plains Cree) filmmaker, creates short films that explore themes of two-spirit experience, gender, sexuality, and madness. Cuthand (n.d.) questions biomedical approaches that dismiss delusions and altered states as meaningless, stating that "even when I am stable and sane, there are things we know and believe as Indigenous people about the beings we share this land with that white people would just scoff at and dismiss" (para 5). Likewise, visual artist Gloria Swain shows that madness is political. Through her work she explores Blackness and madness and how trauma and structural oppression such as racism, sexism, and poverty create madness in Black communities (Swain, 2019). Artists like Cuthand and Swain disrupt the notion of the biomedical model as neutral and objective, expose the racism and colonialism embedded within it, and open up other ways of understanding madness.

Mad art is a way to challenge dominant narratives about madness and Mad people. Art about mental illness, especially when created by non-Mad people, often perpetuates tropes such as a harrowing "descent into madness" (Reid, 2018, para 22) or madness as "mystical creative genius" (Reid, 2018, para 1). Mad art is necessary in order to resist tokenism, fetishization, and tired tropes about madness and Mad people (Reid et al., 2019; Reid, 2018; Walter, 2022).

Importantly, some Mad artists argue against inclusion within the larger arts scene and instead would like to see Mad arts established as its own "undiscipline" led by Mad people (Walter, 2022, para 11). Inclusion runs the risk of neutralizing the political message of Mad art and reverting to problematic tropes and mainstream narratives about recovery from mental illness (Reid, 2018; Walter, 2022). It is crucial to maintain the political, liberationist goals of Mad art. As Reid (2018) states, Mad art is "a way to love, grieve, protest, rage and make change in the world around us. Mad artists … interrupt and disrupt current art spaces and instead create an entirely better future that is necessarily informed by a politics of justice" (para 24).

RESISTING PSYCHIATRIC VIOLENCE, REFRAMING AND RECLAIMING CARE AND TREATMENT

One of Mad Studies' central forms of praxis has been to expose and resist psychiatric violence and create alternative forms of responding to madness, distress, and crisis. Resisting psychiatric violence involves examining, challenging, and reconfiguring concepts of treatment and care. There is a long history and ongoing practice of inflicting violence on those deemed Mad and calling it therapeutic. Terms such as 'treatment' and 'care' can be used euphemistically as a way of eliding violence, perpetuating epistemic injustice, and undermining Mad people's agency (Eales & Peers, 2021; Johnk & Khan, 2019; Scott & Doughty, 2012). Resistance to psychiatric violence takes many forms and the following touches on only a few that expose and resist the violence at the heart of some forms of 'care and treatment' including resistance to coercion, resistance to electroconvulsive therapy (ECT), and the reclamation of care and treatment through the creation of alternatives.

It is important to note that there will always be intra-community disagreement about what constitutes psychiatric violence and what care and treatment should look like. This disagreement even extends to forms of treatment that have a critical mass of people opposed to them, such as ECT and conversion therapy. Correspondingly, within Mad Studies and activism there is much respect for the decisions of individual Mad people and service users to choose biomedical treatments if they so desire. A Mad critique should be understood as a systemic one rather than a recrimination of individual decision making about treatment. For example, individual decisions about taking psychiatric drugs are made within the systemic context of a lack of independent research regarding long-term impacts, among myriad other issues. Not all psychiatric treatment is experienced as bad by all people at all times, however, there are deeply embedded problems with the psy complex. Those who interpret Mad Studies as a value judgement about individual treatment decisions are missing the larger structural picture.

RESISTING COERCIVE CARE: COLONIAL ROOTS

Coercion is foundational to the psy complex because it is built into the very notion of what constitutes care according to the biomedical model. When it is assumed that those deemed mentally ill are incapable of knowing what is best, it follows that 'care' will be paternalistic and coercion will be seen as justifiable. Presumed to be universal, this conceptualization of care is in fact a colonial one that has been violently imposed on Indigenous peoples in an effort to establish settler dominance and erase Indigenous healing practices and ways of knowing (McCreary & Hall, 2024).

Coercive care in the form of forced confinement in asylums in the late 1800s and early 1900s was one technique of settler dominance and land theft (Kanani, 2011; Saisi, 2021; Walker, 2022; Whitt, 2021; Yellow Bird, 2004). For example, Indigenous people in British Columbia in the late 19th and early 20th centuries were forcibly confined in asylums at "a time when the reserve system and federal intervention were at their strongest" (Menzies & Palys, 2006, p. 159). Federal Indian agents, police, and medical professionals sent Indigenous people who were perceived as "troublesome, obdurate, wild, abusive, resistive, or otherwise indecipherable" to asylums far from their communities (p. 161). The confinement of Indigenous people in asylums was not therapeutic, rather, it was a form of social regulation and a means of subjugating Indigenous peoples and ways of knowing, and facilitating land theft (Menzies & Palys, 2006; McCreary & Hall, 2024; Whitt, 2021). For most Indigenous people who were institutionalized, "their committal was effectively a sentence of death" with many never being released and dying of tuberculosis in the institution (Menzies & Palys, 2006, p. 166). Notably, during this time period, Indigenous healing practices were criminalized in an effort to render Indigenous peoples dependent on settler institutions and as a means of establishing colonial "regimes of care," or ways of understanding and responding to 'mental illness' as universal and the only authentic ones (McCreary & Hall, 2024, p. 353).

Some Indigenous people who were institutionalized resisted through refusing to work (perform unpaid labour) at the asylum, refusing food, or refusing to follow the institution's routines. Many also tried to escape, with a small number succeeding. Others resisted through demonstrating assimilation and thereby convincing medical professionals that they were recovered and ready to be released (Menzies & Palys, 2006). Family members also resisted by advocating on behalf of their loved ones by writing to the asylum staff and Indian agents to ask for their return to the community, or by questioning treatment regimes and refusing to sign treatment permission forms (Menzies & Palys, 2006). Resistance and efforts to escape were often pathologized as evidence of illness: "officials pathologized what could be otherwise understood as a reasonable effort to protect one's sense of personal autonomy and self-determination" (McCreary & Hall, 2024, p. 364). Importantly, the attempted eradication of Indigenous healing practices was not totally successful. For example, Witsuwit'en healers still engage in traditional healing practices despite efforts to eradicate them (McCreary & Hall, 2024). Indigenous resistance to the harms of coercive care may involve returning to, or continuing to practice, Indigenous ways of knowing and healing (McCreary & Hall, 2024). Pemina Yellow Bird (2004) emphasizes the crucial role of storytelling in Indigenous resistance to psychiatric violence and the role it plays in returning to Indigenous practices:

> We must then tell our stories of loss, of violation, of what happened to us, and we must at long last grieve those things; we must determine how the past informs us, is part of who we are, and how it walks with us every day of our lives as Native people. We must tell those stories and we must determine for ourselves, based on our own original teachings and instructions, what we must do to care for ourselves.
>
> (p. 3)

Coercive confinement in asylums was also used as a means of containing Black people following the abolition of slavery. For example, Maryland's Hospital for the Negro Insane (later renamed Crownsville) was created in 1910 as a response to what was characterized as increasing rates of "insanity among Negroes who were free. In the view of many prominent physicians at the time, the end of slavery had created a kind of aimless vagrant who needed to be concealed and incarcerated in a new form of institution" (Hylton, 2024, p. 22). White doctors refused to acknowledge the traumatizing impacts of slavery and instead positioned Black people as "infantile at best, or terrors and criminals at worst" (Hylton, 2024, p. 22). Similar to the treatment of Indigenous patients, care for Black asylum patients included unpaid physical labour (Hylton, 2024; Jackson, 2002). Asylum patients, many of whom arrived via police, built the asylum in Maryland from the ground up, and continued to sustain it with their unpaid labour once built. As Hylton (2024) notes, "Crownsville's founding took vestiges of chattel slavery-from the style of the rolls to the financial recordkeeping format used on plantations-and translated them to a clinical setting" (p. 43). Those who were institutionalized at Crownsville resisted by various means including by writing to the local Black newspaper about the abysmal conditions, making escape attempts, and rebelling on the wards (Hylton, 2024).

Similarly, Black patients detained in other asylums also resisted psychiatric violence. For example, Jackson (2002) details a rebellion at the Rusk State hospital in Texas led by a young Black man, Ben Riley, who made "demands for better counseling, organized exercise periods, an end to prisoner beatings, and that all inmates have the same rights enjoyed by the white inmates regarding meals, bathing and freedom of movement" (p. 17). This rebellion involved an attempt to forcibly administer ECT to the hospital superintendent. Similar to Yellow Bird, Jackson (2002) emphasizes the importance of storytelling as a strategy of Black resistance to psychiatric violence:

> The telling of stories has been an integral part of the history of people of African descent... people of African descent have known that our lives and our stories must be spoken, over and over again, so that people will know our truth. History, or at least the official record, is always the history of the dominant group.
>
> (p. 13)

As this discussion begins to show, coercive care is a colonial concept and practice that has been used as a way to extract resources (land and unpaid labour) from Indigenous and Black people and is imbricated with racist assumptions about who is in need of management, confinement, and white control (Brice, 2020; Hylton, 2024; Jackson, 2002; Joseph, 2014; Kanani, 2011; Menzies & Palys, 2006; Roman et al., 2009; Saisi, 2021; Walker, 2015, 2022, Whitt, 2021; Yellow Bird, 2004). Indigenous and Black resistance to psychiatric violence and coercive care has taken many forms over the years, with storytelling being an important form of resistance. It is important for Mad Studies to centre the ways in which psychiatric violence is tied to white supremacy and nation building and to continue to unearth Indigenous and Black narratives and practices of resistance.[1]

CONTEMPORARY RESISTANCE TO COERCIVE CARE

Contemporary examples of formal coercion in mental health care include involuntary institutionalization and hospitalization, locked seclusion, surveillance, mechanical and chemical restraints, involuntary drugging and ECT, and mandatory community treatment such as community treatment orders (CTOs). In many countries, formal coercive practices are regulated by legislation such as Mental Health Acts. Such legislation allows for people to be detained (often colloquially referred to as 'being formed') and/or declared incapable to consent to treatment, and/or manage one's own finances. For example, under the Mental Health Act in Ontario, Canada, a patient who is deemed incompetent will have a substitute decision maker (SDM) appointed; if the patient does not know someone who is able to perform these duties, the Public Guardian and Trustee is made SDM. Being deemed incompetent often hinges on being seen as at risk of harm to oneself and/or others.

Coercion also encompasses informal practices that are not regulated by legislation. For example, in reviewing 161 inpatient charts from a psychiatric hospital in Ontario, Canada

(Daley & Pilling, 2021) we observed countless examples of patients being made to take psychiatric drugs 'with the presence of security.'[2] If a patient expressed resistance (or was perceived as someone who might resist), security guards were called into the room as an informal means of threatening force and coercing compliance. There was frequent documentation of drugs being used to control unwanted behaviours, which can be called "chemical incarceration" (Fabris & Aubrecht, 2014, p. 185). Informal coercion within psychiatric institutions can take many forms including the restriction of 'privileges' such as going outside or accessing a computer or phone, as well as social isolation from family, friends, and other patients, and being kept on locked wards (Berring & Georgaca, 2023; Norvoll & Pederson, 2016). Some patients may agree to 'voluntary' confinement as a means of avoiding involuntary confinement (Beaupert & Brosnan, 2022).

Dominant narratives about coercion in mental health care frame it as justifiable and perpetuate the idea that Mad people need to be managed and controlled, are a danger to self and others, and are unable to act in their own best interest. Those inflicting psychiatric violence (e.g. mental health professionals, institutional security guards) may frame coercive treatment such as restraints as benevolent, necessary, inevitable, as a way of keeping everyone 'safe', or as a response to patient violence (Chapman, 2014; Johnston & Kilty, 2016; Zaheer, 2021).

Mad Studies shows how coercive care is in fact a form of violence, and is not neutral, therapeutic or benevolent (Buck-Zerchin, 2011; Lee-Evoy, 2019; Karanikolas, 2022; Timander, 2020; Wipond, 2024). Mad Studies resists coercion in many forms including the harms of surveillance (Mariette, 2024), restraint, and seclusion (Chapman, 2014; Jacob et al., 2018; Kilty, 2018; Reel, 2019), forced drugging and community treatment orders (Fabris, 2011; Fabris & Aubrecht, 2014), coercive confinement (Bergstresser, 2021; Daya, 2022; Tseris et al., 2022), and carceral intersections (Daley & Radford, 2018; Joseph, 2019; Kilty & Lehalle, 2019; Rembis, 2014; Saisi, 2021). Some Mad scholars explore the law and the United Nation's Convention on the Rights of Persons with

Disabilities as a site of resistance and/or point to the limitations of such (Beaupert & Brosnan, 2022; Logan & Karter, 2022; Minkowitz, 2010; Roper and Gooding, 2018; Shaw, 2022; Sheldon & Spector, 2019; Steele, 2017).

A Mad Studies lens highlights some of the problems with framing psychiatric violence as a response to patient violence and as a means of creating safety. Consider the narrative of a research participant referred to as Ruth in Norvoll and Pederson's (2016) study about coercion in mental health care in Norway:

> When I was forcibly medicated with an injection, there were at least six occasions where I wasn't informed beforehand that I was getting an injection. They just came to the doorway, just like that, those five people standing there with the syringe first. And I got very frightened and tried to defend myself, and was laid down, and I screamed and cried for help. That experience was terrible, and I had great problems afterwards. It was the trauma of my life.
>
> (p. 209)

A Mad Studies lens allows us to surmise that anyone being held down and drugged against their will might, like Ruth, respond with self-defence ('I got very frightened and tried to defend myself') in an effort to break free. Framing self-protection and resistance as 'patient violence' ignores the violence of coercive care that often provokes it (Mckeown et al., 2019). It also ignores the larger structural violence such as poverty, ableism, and colonialism that allow for the existence of the psy complex and lead some to become detained within it. For example, Chapman (2014) points to how these larger structural power relations shaped their experience of committing violence against (restraining and secluding) Indigenous children as a white residential counsellor within the psy complex:

> It was not that we [staff] did not acknowledge that these restraints were traumatic for the children being restrained or for other children witnessing them, but we

were the protagonists in the stories we told and believed. Our violence was only ever a response to their violence. The possibility of imagining their individual violence as a response to our structural, epistemic, *and* individual violence - institutional, disablist, adultist, nationalist, colonialist, and racist - was not available to us. And so because they were the initiators of violence, as we understood it, there was nothing *we* could do to prevent it. We had nothing to do with their violence until it erupted; and our only role was to keep everyone safe.

(p. 24, emphasis in original)

Chapman's narrative reveals that staff did not question the fact that most of the children were Indigenous, while the majority of the staff were white, or see the institution as an outcome and manifestation of colonial violence. Rather, the staff's violence was framed as a response to the children's violence and as a means of keeping everyone safe. This reflects dominant narratives about coercion as a response to patient violence. Chapman's comments about storytelling ('we were the protagonists in the stories we told and believed') also indirectly support the importance of Indigenous and Black storytelling in resisting the racist stories Chapman describes.

A Mad perspective challenges dominant narratives about patient violence and safety and allows for critical questions, such as, what is the context within which patient violence takes place? What violence is inflicted by the psy complex and coercive care? What does self-protection and resistance look like within carceral institutions? Who is made safe by the use of restraints, seclusion, and other forms of coercion, and what lasting harms are inflicted by these practices? Who is more likely to be seen as a 'management problem' in need of coercive care and how does racism and anti-Indigeneity play a role? How does the history of coercion as a colonial tactic influence contemporary psychiatric practices? Who is more likely to be seen as 'bizarre' and in need of coercive intervention and how do transphobia and cisnormativity inform these perceptions?

Framing coercion as a necessary response (rather than as a form of psychiatric violence) to patient violence elides the systemic violence (for example, colonialism, anti-Blackness, and poverty) that results in psychiatric detention as well as the violence of the institution and coerced treatment. A Mad lens shows that these forms of authorized violence are framed as benevolent or necessary while patients are positioned as inherently violent and in need of management and control (Chapman, 2014; Mckeown et al., 2019). These challenges and critical examinations are forms of Mad resistance to psychiatric violence and coercive care.

RESISTING TREATMENT

The biomedical model positions madness as a deficit in need of fixing and as such has invented many forms of treatment over the course of history. One of the main issues with positioning madness as a problem located in individual bodies is that any 'solution' will focus on changing the 'deficient' body, rather than the social conditions that give rise to distress. Many such biomedical treatments have inflicted great harm on the recipients. Some examples include psychosurgery, "an irreversible surgical procedure that permanently destroys healthy brain tissue in order to alter behaviour" the most well-known form being the lobotomy (Reaume, 2008, p. 379). Other examples include insulin-coma therapy, and Metrazol shock, which were precursors to electroconvulsive therapy (Frank, 2002; Weitz, 1988; Whitaker, 2002).

Whether such treatments are seen as therapeutic or become recognized as unjustified violence depends on factors that shift across time and according to context such as sociopolitical conditions, social norms, and prevailing cultural values. It also very much depends on positionality within structural power relations. While some of the treatments named above have fallen out of favour within the psy complex and/or lost credibility within mainstream culture, there were indubitably always people who opposed them and recognized them as forms of violence, but who lacked the social power necessary to effect change (though some may have contributed to the pre-conditions for change). Relatedly, whether such treatments are recognized as unjustified violence also depends on how much value is placed on the lives of the treatment recipients. Once various groups of people are denigrated as sub-human or 'defective' it is easier to garner mass agreement about (or apathy towards) such treatments as therapeutic, deserved, and justified. This is why Mad Studies, in tandem with other anti-oppression frameworks, is valuable as a foundation for resistance; because it counters epistemic injustice, values the lives of denigrated groups, centres lived experience, and has the potential to foster coalitional resistance across identity groups. I use the word *potential* as a means of highlighting that we have not yet seen widespread coalitional efforts that centre Indigenous, Black, racialized, queer, trans, Mad, disabled, and otherwise oppressed voices.

Resistance to ECT is an interesting example to examine in more detail because of its longevity as a psychiatric treatment and because of the sustained Mad resistance to it. As will be seen, part of Mad resistance is in reframing, or maddening, what is presented as objective scientific knowledge and reading against the grain to notice details that are framed as inconsequential, such as the voices and reactions of survivors. The imposition of violence is partially accomplished through language and therefore Mad resistance involves naming violence and the resistance to it as such.

MADDENING THE HISTORY OF ELECTROCONVULSIVE THERAPY

Electroconvulsive Therapy (ECT) was developed by Italian psychiatrist Ugo Cerletti alongside psychiatrist Lucio Bini and was first used on a human being in 1938. This makes ECT a contemporary of the lobotomy, which was also developed in the mid 1930s (Reaume, 2008). While the lobotomy is currently recognized by many as a barbarous form of psychiatric violence, ECT continues to be employed as a psychiatric treatment to this day, including on children (Read, 2023; van

Daalen-Smith et al., 2014).[3] A small minority of countries have banned its use, but it is otherwise still commonly employed. For example, the website for the Centre for Addiction and Mental Health (CAMH) in Toronto, Ontario, proudly proclaims that "each weekday 20 to 25 people receive ECT" as part of their treatment at CAMH (Goldbloom, 2018). ECT was originally characterized as a treatment for schizophrenia, but over time has been touted as a treatment for depression, catatonia, suicidality, bipolar disorder, and obsessive compulsive disorder, amongst others.

ECT involves running an electric current through the brain to cause a grand mal seizure and is usually administered multiple times and repeated over the course of several weeks or months (Burstow, 2016). In its original formulation, ECT was conducted without anaesthetic, commonly caused bone and spinal fractures, and was sometimes fatal (Czech et al., 2020). ECT underwent changes in the 1950s to include the administration of a paralysis-inducing muscle relaxant that reduces (but does not eliminate) the possibility of bone and spinal fractures (Burstow, 2016; Wright, 1990). Other changes include the administration of barbiturates to reduce fear caused by paralysis and changes to the positioning of the electrodes (unilateral as opposed to bitemporal, though both methods continue to be used) (Burstow, 2015, 2016; Wright, 1990). Despite some changes to its administration, the function of ECT remains the same in that it deliberately invokes seizures by running an electrical current through the brain. Many have noted that the desired effect of ECT, much like the lobotomy, has always been to 'treat' patients by causing damage to the brain (Breggin, 2007; Burstow, 2015, 2016). The use of ECT is highly controversial and has been critiqued for causing severe harm to many recipients, including extensive memory loss, cognitive impairment, confusion, loss of motor control, and brain neuropathology (Andre, 2009; Breggin, 1998, 2007; Burstow, 2016; Froede & Baldwin, 1999; Johnstone & Frith, 2005; Mosher & Cohen, 2003).

A brief overview of the history of ECT reveals that it has always been a deeply unethical practice marked by coercion, and was subject to resistance from its inception. Notably, the first human recipient of ECT, referred to in some accounts as S.E., was a criminalized Italian man who did not consent to being experimented upon. S.E. was apprehended by Italian police for being incomprehensible to those around him and boarding a train without a ticket (Frank, 1990). He was sent by police to Cerletti for observation, who deemed him schizophrenic and a suitable test subject for ECT (Frank, 1990). Cerletti and four colleagues administered a first round of ECT using a voltage level that was too low to induce a seizure. Notably, S.E.'s reaction to this first round was recorded as, "non una seronda! mortifera! ('not again it will kill me!')" (Wright, 1990, p. 71). Nevertheless, Cerletti proceeded with a second round using higher voltage, against S.E.'s wishes and against the consensus in the room (Wright, 1990). This second round induced a seizure and was characterized as a success by the psychiatrists (Wright, 1990). S.E. was alleged to have been "in remission" following 13 subsequent ECT treatments over the course of two months and by some accounts was "lost to follow up" after two years (Wright, 1990, p. 72).[4]

While we do not have a first-person account from S.E., we can use a Mad Studies lens to interpret what doctors referred to as becoming 'lost to follow up' as a possible form of resistance. In other words, S.E. may have mercifully escaped further non-consensual experimentation at the hands of these psychiatrists. Likewise, a Mad Studies framework helps us understand that what was done to S.E. cannot reasonably be called 'treatment,' when in fact it was non-consensual medical experimentation. While much of the historical and medical literature characterizes what happened to S.E. as treatment for schizophrenia, there should be no argument that this was unethical coerced experimentation (rather than simply 'treatment' or 'human trials'), given that the effect on humans was entirely unknown, and the recipient was coerced. Mad Studies allows us to recognize violence and notice resistance to it rather than glossing over S.E.'s response ("not again it will kill me!") as an inconsequential detail. Likewise, it is important to notice and highlight that S.E. was criminalized and pathologized because this means that he was at higher risk of falling victim to the punitive power of the state and of being seen as deserving of what befell him.

The history of ECT does not stop with S.E. and reveals further disturbing and violent uses of ECT across many contexts. Following the supposed success of the experimentation inflicted on S.E., ECT rapidly gained popularity across Europe, the United States, and eventually in Canada for treating people with all kinds of psychiatric diagnoses including depression and bipolar disorder. This rapid proliferation of ECT was linked to its use in Nazi Germany and the Nazis' influence across Europe in the 1940s. A few years after its introduction in Italy, a form of ECT that was modified to increase its fatal effect was used in Nazi Germany to kill hospitalized psychiatric patients in a eugenic bid to reduce the number of people in psychiatric institutions and increase the number of hospital beds for injured soldiers (Czech et al., 2020; Gazdag et al., 2017). ECT was also used at Auschwitz in criminal experimentation on those imprisoned there, many of whom died during ECT. The spread of ECT in the United States is also linked to Nazi Germany; one of the first major proponents of ECT in the United States was there as a means of escaping anti-Semitism in Europe (Czech et al., 2020).

ECT continued to be used for other nefarious purposes. In the 1950s and 1960s, psychiatric patients were non-consensual, unwitting, subjects in brainwashing experiments funded by the Canadian government and the American Central Intelligence Agency (CIA).[5] These experiments, referred to as project MK-ULTRA, were conducted by Dr Ewen Cameron at the Allen Memorial Institute, located at McGill University in Montreal, Quebec. Patients were subjected to high levels of ECT, drugs, sensory deprivation, and induced comas in an effort to achieve mind control (Shephard et al., 2020; Gold, 2022). Canadian and American governments and McGill University have failed to accept liability and apologize for the lasting damage inflicted, despite victims' continued quest for such (Shephard et al., 2020). Of note, Dr. Cameron's experiments have also been linked to contemporary torturous interrogation techniques employed at Guantanamo Bay in the 'war on terror' (Shephard et al., 2020).

Though more research is needed to uncover the details, there are indications that ECT may have been used in sanatoriums (known as Indian hospitals) as part of non-consensual medical experimentation inflicted on Indigenous people in Canada in the 1950s (Carreiro, 2017; Geddes, 2017; Humphrey, 2017). ECT has also been used on 2SLGBTQI people as a technology of conversion therapy, a violent practice that aims to transform queer and trans people into cisgender heterosexuals (Blakemore, 2023; Kinitz et al., 2022; Salway & Ashley, 2022).

Despite ECT's sordid history in Nazi Germany, and its use in non-consensual human experimentation and conversion therapy, ECT has survived as a psychiatric treatment to the present day. Some have pointed out that ECT is used more frequently on women, particularly those who are elderly, due to sexism and misogyny (Burstow, 2006; van Daalen-Smith, 2011, 2015). ECT continues to be a deeply troubling and ethically suspect practice marked by continued failures to obtain true informed consent from its recipients, even in cases when its use is 'voluntary.' Women have been especially subject to these failures (Burstow, 2016; Clarke et al., 2018; Ejaredar & Hagen, 2014; van Daalen-Smith, 2011, 2015).

CONTEMPORARY ORGANIZED RESISTANCE TO ELECTROCONVULSIVE THERAPY

ECT has been subject to longstanding and ongoing organized resistance efforts. In Ontario, such organized Mad resistance dates back to at least 1983 and has taken the shape of direct action, and advocacy to change policy and legislation (Weitz, 2018). For example, in the early 1980s, survivors came together to form the Ontario Coalition to Stop Electroshock. In 1984, this coalition held public hearings on ECT at Toronto City Hall during which 18 people who experienced ECT and 19 friends and family members of people who experienced ECT testified as to their experiences (Froede & Baldwin, 1999). These hearings were groundbreaking in that they centred the voices of people with lived experience, a rare occurrence given that the perspectives of professionals are usually prioritized (Froede & Baldwin, 1999). A content analysis of the survivors' testimonies identified common themes including lasting debilitating after-effects, inadequate information sharing about ECT and its effects, and questionable practices in acquiring consent for treatment. The analysis also found that "feelings of degradation and dehumanisation were strongly represented in the testimonies" and concluded that ECT should be banned (Froede & Baldwin, 1999, p. 187). Excerpts from the testimonies include harrowing first-person accounts of ECT treatment such as the following:

> I lay there paralysed trying desperately just to move a finger to let them know that I was still there so they wouldn't turn the electricity on because I had heard from one of the other young guys on the ward that it really hurts [and] I felt like I was dying every time one of them was administered.
>
> (Froede & Baldwin, 1999, p. 184)

These public hearings were part of a bigger effort to acquire a moratorium on ECT in Ontario, spearheaded by psychiatric survivor, activist, and politician David Reville (Reville & Church, 2012). Efforts to obtain the moratorium were ultimately unsuccessful, largely due to the privileging of the perspectives of psychiatric professionals (Neil, 2021; Weitz, 2018). However, activists continued the fight against ECT. The Ontario Coalition to Stop Electroshock became Resistance Against Psychiatry in 1989 and eventually reformed as the Coalition Against Psychiatric Assault (CAPA) in 2003 (Weitz, 2018). CAPA held public hearings at Toronto City Hall in 2005, similar to the hearings held in 1984 (Burstow, 2015). A report summarizing these hearings found that many of the issues identified in 1984 persist, such as the use of coercion, lack of informed consent, experiences of fear, humiliation, and trauma during treatment, and lasting debilitating effects (Electroshock is not a Healing Option, 2005). For example, a participant pseudonymously referred to as Paivi who received 30 shock treatments stated, "chunks of my memory are missing, a part of my being has been wiped away" and "I used to be able to use my imagination to paint... this extreme treatment has numbed my emotions. The numbed emotions continue today. I've never been able to connect. It's as if I'm looking through a window watching" (p. 12). The report lists a number of recommendations including the use of non-medical, community-based treatment methods and the banning of ECT.

In addition to these public hearings, activists have engaged in direct action such as sit-ins and protests at government offices, hospitals, clinics, and meetings of the American Psychiatric Association (Weitz, 2018). The 2000s have seen numerous 'Stop Shocking Our Mothers and Grandmothers' protests taking place on Mother's Day (Weitz, 2018). In 2010, a member of Provincial Parliament representing the Ontario New Democrat Party, Cheri DiNovo, put forward a bill to end the public funding of ECT, but the bill was not called for debate (Bill 67, Ending Public Funding of Electroconvulsive Therapy Act). CAPA remains active and continues to fight against ECT (https://coalitionagainstpsychiatricassault.wordpress.com).

This brief history of ECT and some of the resistance to it is instructive in thinking about the need for coalitional Mad resistance. A Mad Studies lens illuminates ECT as a practice haunted by non-consensual violent experimentation from its first human recipient onwards. Despite at least 40 years of Mad resistance to ECT, it is still commonly declared by medical professionals to be safe and effective and continues to be employed (Levine, 2004; Maylea & Daya, 2019). Due to advocacy, changing social norms, and other sociopolitical factors, practices such as brainwashing, non-consensual human experimentation, conversion therapy, and concentration camps have been, to varying degrees, recognized in some countries as forms of violence.[6] What if everyone who opposes non-consensual human experimentation, concentration camps, brainwashing, and conversion therapy were also united in their opposition to the specific technologies employed therein, such as ECT? What could a large-scale, coalitional resistance to ECT look like? These are important questions to consider in the ongoing fight against ECT.

RECLAIMING TREATMENT AND CREATING ALTERNATIVES

In addition to direct action as described above, Mad resistance also takes the shape of creating alternatives outside of mental health systems. At the heart of many of these alternatives is the practice of peer support. Peer support assumes that those with lived experience of distress and mental health systems are uniquely situated to provide support to others in similar situations (Davidow & Akiva, 2023; Faulkner, 2017). Peer support practices have long existed in communities who are unsupported or harmed by social services including racialized, queer, trans, and otherwise oppressed communities (Kaufman-Mthimkhulu, 2020). Peer support can be seen as working towards epistemic justice in that it supports agency and self-determination and believes people about the nature of their experiences and how they would like to respond to them.

Peer support can take many forms. For example, peer-led Hearing Voices groups provide a place for those who hear voices to meet and share experiences without judgment and without applying a pathologizing lens (Dillon & Longden, 2013). Whereas the content of what voices say is often disregarded as meaningless and a pathological symptom of illness, the Hearing Voices approach restores social context by making links between voice hearing and traumatic experiences such as childhood abuse (Corstens & Longden, 2013). Many organized peer support services are engaged in advocacy and embrace non-medical and non-carceral approaches that do not rely on police and mental health professionals. For example, Project Lets (United States) provides peer support services that are non-carceral and is a peer-led organization committed to collective liberation and community-based responses to distress (Kaufman-Mthimkhulu, 2020). Likewise, Trans Lifeline (Canada/United States) is a peer support suicide hotline that, unlike most such services (Wipond, 2023), does not use non-consensual active rescue. Trans Lifeline does not call emergency responders or police unless requested because police intervention and involuntary hospitalization can lead to discrimination in psychiatric hospitals, increased suicidality, and the denial of future gender-affirming care (Trans Lifeline, 2020). In addition to providing alternatives to medical treatment in the form of peer support services, many grassroots peer-led initiatives create new knowledge about distress, crisis, and experiences of madness, and develop trainings. For example, the Wildflower Alliance (United States) offers peer support services as well as training on anti-oppression and alternatives to hospitalization, and the Fireweed Collective (United States) has created a crisis toolkit (https://fireweedcollective.org/crisis-toolkit/).

PEER SUPPORT: TROUBLES WITH CO-OPTION

In the Global North, peer support workers have been integrated into mental health systems. Growing interest in incorporating peer support into the psy complex raises thorny questions about what happens when people with lived experience are employed in peer support roles within these systems (Faulkner, 2017; Scott & Doughty, 2012; Voronka, 2016, 2017, 2019). These include questions about representational authority, or who should speak for whom (Voronka, 2016), as well as what happens when peer support becomes a commodity and a precarious form of employment within neoliberal mental health systems (Voronka, 2017). Peer workers risk becoming assimilated into psy systems as para-professionals who encourage self-governance and compliance with biomedical approaches (Voronka, 2017). The integration of peer support into mental health services can remove it from its experiential knowledge base, thereby co-opting and neutralizing it (Faulkner, 2017).

Peer support's troubles with co-optation also raises questions about whether meaningful change can be accomplished from within, or whether the focus should be on creating change outside of the psy complex. Making improvements to the psy complex can increase its capacity to reproduce itself and perpetuate harms (Burstow, 2014). In other words, "instead of making the system more just, it spreads an unjust system to more people" (Ben-Moshe, 2020, p. 16). At the same time, there are many Mad people who engage (both freely and coerced) with the psy complex and there is much that could be done to address harms from within mental health systems. As with most binaries, an either-or approach is likely unhelpful. However, it is important to be wary of the ways in which grassroots and liberationist approaches and practices can be co-opted and become far removed from the interests of the people who initially created them.

This chapter has provided a partial account of Mad Studies as praxis, or in other words, what Mad Studies can help us do. In concluding this chapter, I emphasize that it is crucial to recognize that epistemic injustice works to invalidate resistance to the psy complex by those deemed in need of its interventions. Psychiatric constructs such as 'insight' are used to pathologize resistance to psychiatric treatment (Pilling et al., 2018; Rivest, 2022). Resistance to treatment is construed as lack of insight into illness and as further proof of 'mental illness,' especially for racialized, poor, queer, and trans people (Pilling et al., 2018). Those currently ensnared in the psy complex are easily dismissed as too ill, incompetent, and disconnected from reality to know what is best for them. The voices of psychiatric survivors and people with lived experience who resist or critique harmful psychiatric and carceral practices continue to be positioned as biased, invalid, irrational, too emotional, and polemical (Johnstone & Frith, 2005; Kilty & Orsini, 2024; Mayfield & Daya, 2019). This underscores the importance of Mad praxis as a means of achieving epistemic justice through the reclamation and honouring of Mad knowledge and ways of being. It also points to the essential nature of coalitional action and allyship in ending iatrogenic harms and violent treatment. As the popularized Chilean protest chant goes, 'the people, united, will never be defeated.'

Recommended resources

Joseph, A. J. (2019). Contemporary forms of legislative imprisonment and colonial violence in forensic mental health. In A. Daley, L. Costa, & P. Beresford (Eds.), *Madness, violence, and power: A critical collection* (pp. 169–183). University of Toronto Press. https://doi.org/10.3138/9781442629981-017

Kalathil, J. (2013). 'Hard to reach'? Racialized groups and mental health service user involvement. In P. Staddon (Ed.), *Mental health service users in research: Critical sociological perspectives* (pp. 121–133). Policy Press. https://doi.org/10.1332/policypress/9781447307334.003.0009

Snyder, S. N., Pitt, K. A., Shanouda, F., Voronka, J., Reid, J., & Landry, D. (2019). Unlearning through Mad Studies: Disruptive pedagogical praxis. *Curriculum Inquiry, 49*(4), 485–502. https://doi.org/10.1080/03626784.2019.1664254

Weitz, D. (2018). *Resistance matters: The radical vision of an antipsychiatry activist.* Mad in America. www.madinamerica.com/wp-content/uploads/2019/06/Resistance-Matters-April-2019.pdf

NOTES

1 For a digital exhibition of documents pertaining to the treatment of Black, Indigenous, poor, and immigrant people in American 19th-century asylums, see the *Race, class, and mental health* section of the website entitled, *Hearing voices: Memoirs from the margins of mental health* created by the Library Company of Philadelphia: https://librarycompany.org/hearingvoices-online/section4.html

2 'Medication administered with the presence of security' is the language often used in psychiatric charts, which is a passive formulation that removes the agent from the sentence and linguistically neutralizes what is often a traumatizing event.

3 There are, unsurprisingly, contemporary apologists for the lobotomy as well as advocates for psychosurgery more broadly. Reaume (2008) notes that the history of lobotomy continues under other names in that psychosurgeries

(cingulotomy and capsulotomy) are on the rise in North America (see also Wipond, 2024).

4 There are conflicting accounts of the treatment of S. E. including the exact timelines of his 'treatment,' who was present when S. E. was first experimented upon, and whether S. E. was 'lost to follow up' or suffered further experimentation. Wright (1990), who I draw upon here, cites Cerletti's writing as his source, amongst others.

5 It is possible that this practice began in the late 1940s but the exact start date is unknown. Likewise, the total number of victims/survivors and complete list of victim/survivor names have never been released (Shephard et al., 2020).

6 Mainstream recognition of such practices as violent is tenuous, incomplete, and never guaranteed. For example, conversion therapy still takes place in many places including Canada despite its recent criminalization (Sampson et al., 2022).

REFERENCES

Abdillahi, I., Meerai, S., & Poole, J. (2017). When the suffering is compounded: Towards anti-Black sanism. In S. Wehbi & H. Parada (Eds.), *Reimagining anti-oppression social work practice* (pp. 109–122). Canadian Scholars Press.

Andre, L. (2009). *Doctors of deception: What they don't want you to know about shock treatment.* Rutgers University Press. https://doi.org/10.36019/9780813546520

Archibald, L. (2024). Maintaining the fidelity of Mad Studies (An ode to Mad Studies 2). *Asylum, 31*(1), 16–17.

Armstrong, V. & LeFrançois, B. A. (2022). Interrogating Mad Studies in the academy: Bridging the community/academy divide. In P. Beresford & J. Russo (Eds.), *The Routledge international handbook of Mad Studies* (pp. 315–326). Routledge. https://doi.org/10.4324/9780429465444-37

Ballantyne, E., Maclean, K., Collie, S. A., Deeming, L., & Fraser, E. (2020). Mad people's history and identity: A Mad Studies critical pedagogy project. In *Public sociology as educational practice* (pp. 25–36). Bristol University Press. https://doi.org/10.1332/policypress/9781529201406.003.0003

Beaupert, F. & Brosnan, L. (2022). Weaponizing absent knowledges: Countering the violence of mental health law. In P. Beresford & J. Russo (Eds.), *The Routledge international handbook of Mad Studies* (pp. 119–133). Routledge. https://doi.org/10.4324/9780429465444-17

Begum, N. (2006). *Doing it for themselves: Participation and black and minority ethnic service users.* Social Care Institute for Excellence. https://lx.iriss.org.uk/content/scie-report-14-doing-it-themselves-participation-and-black-and-minority-ethnic-service-users.html

Ben-Moshe, L., Cory, R. C., Feldbaum, M., & Sagendorf, K. (Eds.). (2005). *Building pedagogical curb cuts: Incorporating disability in the university classroom and curriculum.* The Graduate School, Syracuse University.

Ben-Moshe, L. (2020). *Decarcerating disability: Deinstitutionalization and prison abolition.* University of Minnesota Press. https://doi.org/10.5749/j.ctv10vm2vw

Beresford, P. & Rose, R. (2009). Chapter two: Background. In P. Beresford, A. Faulkner, A. Sweeney, D. Rose, & M. Nettle (Eds.), *This is survivor research* (pp. 11–21). PCCS Books.

Beresford, P. & Wallcraft, J. (1997). Psychiatric system survivors and emancipatory research: Issues, overlaps and differences. In C. Barnes & G. Mercer, *Doing disability research* (pp. 66–87). Disability Press.

Bergstresser, S. M. (2021). Involuntary psychiatric commitment in the era of COVID-19: Systemic social oppression and discourses of risk in public health and bioethics. *International Journal of Critical Diversity Studies*, 4(1), 92–106. https://doi.org/10.13169/intercritdivestud.4.1.0092

Berring, L. L. & Georgaca, E. (2023). A call for transformation: Moving away from coercive measures in mental health care. *Healthcare*, 11(16), 2315–2318. www.doi.org/10.3390/healthcare11162315

Blakey, H. (2005). *Participation – why bother? The views of black and minority ethnic mental health service users on participation in the NHS in Bradford.* International Centre for Participation Studies, University of Bradford. https://bradscholars.brad.ac.uk/handle/10454/3798

Breggin, P. R. (1998). Electroshock: Scientific, ethical, and political issues. *International Journal of Risk & Safety in Medicine*, 11(1), 5–40.

Breggin, P. R. (2007). *Brain-disabling treatments in psychiatry: Drugs, electroshock, and the psychopharmaceutical complex.* Springer Publishing Company.

Bill 67, *Ending Public Funding of Electroconvulsive Therapy Act*, 2nd Session, 29th Legislature, 2010.

Blakemore, E. (2023, August 23). *Gay conversion therapy's disturbing 19th-century origins*. History. www.history.com/news/gay-conversion-therapy-origins-19th-century

Brice, A. (2020, November 19). *How the U.S. government created an "insane asylum" to imprison Native Americans.* UC Berkley News. https://news.berkeley.edu/2020/11/19/using-disability-to-imprison-native-americans/

Buck-Zerchin, D. (2011). Seventy years of coercion in psychiatric institutions, experienced and witnessed. In T. W. Kallert, J. E. Mezzich, & J. Monahan (Eds.), *Coercive treatment in psychiatry: Clinical, legal and ethical aspects* (pp. 235–243). Wiley-Blackwell. https://doi.org/10.1002/9780470978573.ch14

Burstow, B. (2003). From pills to praxis: Psychiatric survivors and adult education. *Canadian Journal for the Study of Adult Education, 17*(1), 1–18. https://doi.org/10.56105/cjsae.v17i1.1868

Burstow, B. (2006). Electroshock as a form of violence against women. *Violence Against Women, 12*(4), 372–392. https://doi.org/10.1177/1077801206286404

Burstow, B. (2014). The withering away of psychiatry: An attrition model for antipsychiatry. In B. Burstow, B. A. LeFrançois, & S. Diamond (Eds.), *Psychiatry disrupted: Theorizing resistance and crafting the (r)evolution* (pp. 34–51). McGill-Queen's University Press. https://doi.org/10.1515/9780773590304-006

Burstow, B. (2015). *Psychiatry and the business of madness: An ethical and epistemological accounting.* Palgrave Macmillan. https://doi.org/10.1057/9781137503855

Burstow, B. (2016). Legitimating damage and control: The ethicality of electroshock research. *Intersectionalities: A global journal of social work analysis, research, polity, and practice, 5*(1), 94–109. https://doi.org/10.48336/IJVZIY2850

de Bie, A. (2019). Finding ways (and words) to move: Mad student politics and practices of loneliness. *Disability & Society, 34*(7–8), 1154–1179. https://doi.org/10.1080/09687599.2019.1609910

de Bie, A. (2022). Respectfully distrusting "students as partners" practice in higher education: Applying a Mad politics of partnership. *Teaching in Higher Education*, 27(6), 717–737. https://doi.org/10.1080/13562517.2020.1736023

de Bie, A., Marquis, E., Cook-Sather, A., & Luqueño, L. P. (2019). Valuing knowledge(s) and cultivating confidence: Contributions of student-faculty pedagogical partnerships to epistemic justice. In J. Hoffman, P. Blessinger, & M. Makhanya (Eds.), *Strategies for fostering inclusive classrooms in higher education: International perspectives on equity and inclusion* (pp. 35–48). Emerald Publishing Limited. https://doi.org/10.1108/s2055-364120190000016004

Carette, L., de Bie, L., Brown, K., & De Schauwer, E. (2024). Keeping the conversation going: Rendering each other capable while creating zines. *Qualitative Inquiry*. https://doi.org/10.1177/10778004241253263

Carr, S. (2022). Institutional ceremonies? The (im)possibilities of transformative co-production in mental health. In P. Beresford & J. Russo (Eds.), *The Routledge international handbook of Mad Studies* (pp. 142–153). Routledge. https://doi.org/10.4324/9780429465444-20

Carr, S. (2015). Individual narratives and collective experience: Capturing lesbian, gay and bisexual service user experiences. In P. Staddon (Ed.), *Mental health service users in research: Critical sociological perspectives* (pp. 135–151). Policy Press. https://doi.org/10.1332/policypress/9781447307334.003.0010

Carreiro, D. (2017, September 22). "Our people were experimented on": *Indigenous sanatorium survivors recall medical tests.* CBC News. www.cbc.ca/news/canada/manitoba/indigenous-sanatorium-suvivors-medical-experiments-1.4301131

Castrodale, M. A. (2017). Critical disability studies and mad studies: Enabling new pedagogies in practice. *Canadian Journal for the study of Adult Education*, 29(1), 49–66. https://doi.org/10.56105/cjsae.v29i1.5357

Castrodale, M. A. (2019). Mad Studies and mad–positive music. *New Horizons in Adult Education and Human Resource*

Development, *31*(1), 40–58. https://doi.org/10.1002/nha3. 20239

Cea-Madrid, J. C. & Castillo-Parada, T. (2021). Enloqueciendo la academia: Estudios Locos, metodologías críticas e investigación militante en salud mental. *Revista Latinoamericana de Metodología de las Ciencias Sociales*, *11*(2), 1–11. https://doi.org/10.24215/18537863e097

Chapman, C. (2014). Becoming perpetrator: How I came to accept restraining and confining disabled Aboriginal children. In B. Burstow, B. A. LeFrançois, & S. Diamond (Eds.), *Psychiatry disrupted: Theorizing resistance and crafting the (r)evolution* (pp. 16–33). McGill-Queen's University Press. https://doi.org/10.1515/9780773590304-005

Chandler, E. (2019). Introduction: Cripping the arts in Canada. *Canadian Journal of Disability Studies*, *8*(1), 1–14. https://doi.org/10.15353/cjds.v8i1.468

Church, K. (2013). Making madness matter in academic practice. In B.A. LeFrançois, R. Menzies, & G. Reaume, *Mad matters: A critical reader in Canadian Mad Studies* (pp. 181–190). Canadian Scholars Press.

Church, K. (2015). "It's complicated": Blending disability and Mad Studies in the corporatising university. In H. Spandler, J. Anderson, & B. Sapey (Eds.), *Madness, distress and the politics of disablement* (pp. 261–270). Policy Press. https://doi.org/10.46692/9781447314592.020

Clarke, K. A., Barnes, M., & Ross, D. (2018). I had no other option: Women, electroconvulsive therapy, and informed consent. *International Journal of Mental Health Nursing*, *27*(3), 1077–1085. https://doi.org/10.1111/inm.12420

Cohen, B. M. (2016). *Psychiatric hegemony: A Marxist theory of mental illness*. Palgrave Macmillan. https://doi.org/10.1057/978-1-137-46051-6

Corstens, D. & Longden, E. (2013). The origins of voices: Links between life history and voice hearing in a survey of 100 cases. *Psychosis*, *5*(3), 270–285. https://doi.org/10.1080/17522439.2013.816337

Costa, L. & Ross, L. (2023). Mad Studies genealogy and praxis. *International Mad Studies Journal*, *1*(1), e1–8. https://doi. org/10.58544/imsj.v1i1.5239

Cuthand, T. J. (n.d.). *Spotlight on Madness by Thirza Cuthand*. Akimbo. https://akimbo.ca/akimblog/spotlight-on-madness-by-thirza-cuthand/

Czech, H., Ungvari, G. S., Uzarczyk, K., Weindling, P., & Gazdag, G. (2020). Electroconvulsive therapy in the shadow of the gas chambers: Medical innovation and human experimentation in Auschwitz. *Bulletin of the History of Medicine*, *94*(2), 244–266. https://doi.org/10.1353/bhm.2020.0036

Daley, A. & Radford, K. (2018). Queer and trans incarceration distress: Considerations from a mad queer abolitionist perspective. In A. Mills & K. Kendall (Eds.), *Mental health in prisons: Critical perspectives on treatment and confinement* (pp. 285–307). Palgrave Macmillan. https://doi.org/1 0.1007/978-3-319-94090-8_12

Daley, A. & Pilling, M. D. (2021). Introduction: Psychiatric documentation, power, and violence. In A. Daley & M. D. Pilling (Eds.), *Interrogating psychiatric narratives of madness: Documented lives* (pp. 1–31). Palgrave Macmillan. https://doi.org/10.1007/978-3-030-83692-4_1

Davidow, S. & Akiva, E. (2023, March 31). *LGBTQIA+ peer respites: The personal is political*. Mad in America. www. madinamerica.com/2023/03/lgbtqia-peer-respites/

Davies, A. W. (2023). Maddening pre-service early childhood education and care through poetics: Dismantling epistemic injustice through mad autobiographical poetics. *Contemporary Issues in Early Childhood*, *24*(2), 124–146. https://doi. org/10.1177/14639491231155555

Davies, A. (2022). Professional ruptures in pre-service ECEC: Maddening early childhood education and care. *Curriculum Inquiry*, *52*(5), 571–592. https://doi.org/10.1080/03626784. 2022.2149027

Davar, B. V. (2015). Identity constructions for 'mentally disturbed' women: Identities versus institutions. In B. Davar & T. K. S. Ravindran (Eds.), *Gendering mental health: Knowledges, identities and institutions* (pp. 193–219). New

Delhi: Oxford University Press. https://doi.org/10.1093/acp rof:oso/9780199453535.003.0009

Daya, I. (2022). Russian dolls and epistemic crypts: A lived experience reflection on epistemic injustice and psychiatric confinement. *Incarceration*, 3(2). https://doi.org/10.1177/26326663221103445

Dillon, J. & Longden, E. (2013). Hearing voices groups: Creating safe spaces to share taboo experiences. In M. Romme & S. Escher (Eds.), *Psychosis as a personal crisis: An experience-based approach* (pp. 129–139). Routledge. https://doi.org/10.4324/9780203696682

Doharty, N. (2024). Can Black critical theory sit with Mad Studies in education in Britain? *Pedagogy, Culture & Society*, 1–16. https://doi.org/10.1080/14681366.2024.2366287

Eales, L. & Peers, D. (2021). Care haunts, hurts, heals: The promiscuous poetics of queer crip Mad care. *Journal of Lesbian Studies*, 25(3), 163–181. https://doi.org/10.1080/10894160.2020.1778849

Ejaredar, M. & Hagen, B. (2014). I was told it restarts your brain: Knowledge, power, and women's experiences of ECT. *Journal of Mental Health*, 23(1), 31–37. https://doi.org/10.3109/09638237.2013.841870

Coalition Against Psychiatric Assault, Electroshock Panel. (2005). *Electroshock is not a healing option: The report of the Panel.* https://coalitionagainstpsychiatricassault.wordpress.com/wp-content/uploads/2010/09/shockreport.pdf

Fabris, E. (2011). *Tranquil prisons: Chemical incarceration under community treatment orders.* University of Toronto Press. https://doi.org/10.3138/9781442696884

Fabris, E. & Aubrecht, K. (2014). Chemical constraint: Experiences of psychiatric coercion, restraint, and detention as carceratory techniques. In Ben-Mosche, L. (Ed.), *Disability incarcerated: Imprisonment and disability in the United States and Canada* (pp. 185–199). Palgrave Macmillan. https://doi.org/10.1057/9781137388476_10

Faulkner, A. (2004). *The ethics of survivor research: Guidelines for the ethical conduct of research carried out by mental health service users and survivors.* Policy Press.

Faulkner, A. (2017). Survivor research and Mad Studies: the role and value of experiential knowledge in mental health research. *Disability & Society*, *32*(4), 500–520. https://doi.org/10.1080/09687599.2017.1302320

Faulkner, A. (2021). Knowing our own minds: Transforming the knowledge base of madness and distress. In R. Ellis, S. Kendal, & S. J. Taylor (Eds.), *Voices in the history of madness: Personal and professional perspectives on mental health and illness* (pp. 333–357). Springer International Publishing. https://doi.org/10.1007/978-3-030-69559-0_16

Frank, L. R. (2002). Electroshock: A crime against the spirit. *Ethical Human Sciences and Services*, *4*(1), 63–71.

Frank, L. R. (1990). Electroshock: death, brain damage, memory loss, and brainwashing. *The Journal of Mind and Behavior*, *11*(3/4), 489–512.

Freire, P. (1972). *Education for critical consciousness.* Seabury Press.

Froede, E. & Baldwin, S. (1999) Toronto public hearings on electroshock: Testimonies of ECT survivors – Review and content analysis. *International Journal of Risk & Safety in Medicine*, *12*(1999), 181–192.

Gazdag, G., Ungvari, G. S., & Czech, H. (2017). Mass killing under the guise of ECT: The darkest chapter in the history of biological psychiatry. *History of Psychiatry*, *28*(4), 482–488. https://doi.org/10.1177/0957154x17724037

Geddes, G. (2017). *Medicine unbundled: A journey through the minefields of Indigenous health care.* Heritage House.

Gold, E. (2022). *Tracing eugenics: The rise of totalizing psychiatric ideology in Canada* [Doctoral Dissertation, University of Toronto]. TSpace Repository.

Goldbloom, D. (2018, April 11). *The past, present and future of electroconvulsive therapy.* Centre for Addiction and Mental Health. www.camh.ca/en/camh-news-and-stories/the-past-present-and-future-of-electroconvulsive-therapy#:~:text=The%20benefits%20of%20ECT%20led,and%20in%20Toronto%20by%201941.

Humphreys, M. (2017, March 14). *B.C. author tells the horrific story of so-called "Indian hospitals".* CBC News. www.

cbc.ca/news/canada/british-columbia/hospital-indigenous-author-1.4024075

Hylton, A. (2024). *Madness: Race and insanity in a Jim Crow asylum*. Grand Central Publishing.

Jacob, J. D., Homes, D., Rioux, D., & Corneau, P. (2018). Patients' perspective on mechanical restraints in acute and emergency psychiatric settings: A poststructural feminist analysis. In J. Kilty & E. Dej (Eds.), *Containing madness: Gender and 'psy' in institutional contexts* (pp. 93–117). Palgrave Macmillan. https://doi.org/10.1007/978-3-319-89749-3_5

Jackson, V. (2002). In our own voice: African-American stories of oppression, survival and recovery in mental health systems. *International Journal of Narrative Therapy and Community Work, 2*, 11–31.

Johnk, L. & Khan, S. A. (2019). "Cripping the fuck out": A queer crip mad manifesta against the medical industrial complex. *Feral Feminisms*, 9, 27–38.

Johnston, M. S. & Kilty, J. M. (2016). "It's for their own good": Techniques of neutralization and security guard violence against psychiatric patients. *Punishment & Society*, *18*(2), 177–197. https://doi.org/10.1177/1462474516635884

Johnstone, L. & Frith, H. (2005). Discourse analysis and the experience of ECT. *Psychology and Psychotherapy: Theory, Research and Practice, 78*(2), 189–203. https://doi.org/10.1348/147608305x26657

Jones, N., Harrison, J., Aguiar, R., & Munro, L. (2014). Transforming research for transformative change in mental health: Towards the future. In G. Nelson, B. Kloos, & J. Ornelas (Eds.), *Community psychology and community mental health: Towards transformative change* (pp. 351–372). Oxford University Press. https://doi.org/10.1093/acprof:oso/9780199362424.003.0017

Jordan, J. T. & McNiel, D. E. (2020). Perceived coercion during admission into psychiatric hospitalization increases risk of suicide attempts after discharge. *Suicide and Life-Threatening Behavior, 50*(1), 180–188. https://doi.org/10.1111/sltb.12560

Joseph, A. J. (2014). A prescription for violence: The legacy of colonization in contemporary forensic mental health and the production of difference. *Critical Criminology, 22*, 273–292. https://doi.org/10.1007/s10612-013-9208-1

Joseph, A. J. (2019). Contemporary forms of legislative imprisonment and colonial violence in forensic mental health. In A. Daley, L. Costa, & P. Beresford (Eds.), *Madness, violence, and power: A critical collection* (pp. 169–183). University of Toronto Press. https://doi.org/10.3138/9781442629981-017

Kafai, S. (2021). *Crip kinship: The disability justice and art activism of Sins Invalid*. Arsenal Pulp Press.

Kafer, A. (2013). *Feminist, queer, crip*. Indiana University Press.

Kalathil, J. & Jones, N. (2016). Unsettling disciplines: Madness, identity, research, knowledge. *Philosophy, Psychiatry, & Psychology, 23*(3), 183–188. https://doi.org/10.1353/ppp.2016.0016

Kalathil, J. (2009). *Dancing to our own tunes: Reassessing black and minority ethnic mental health service user involvement*. National Survivor User Network.

Kalathil, J. (2011). *Dancing to our own tunes: Reprint of the 2008 report with a review of work undertaken to take the recommendations forward*. National Survivor User Network.

Kalathil, J. (2013). "Hard to reach"? Racialized groups and mental health service user involvement. In P. Staddon (Ed.), *Mental health service users in research: Critical sociological perspectives* (pp. 121–133). Policy Press. https://doi.org/10.1332/policypress/9781447307334.003.0009

Kanani, N. (2011). Race and madness: Locating the experiences of racialized people with psychiatric histories in Canada and the United States. *Critical Disability Discourse, 3*, 1–14. https://cdd.journals.yorku.ca/index.php/cdd/article/view/31564

Karanikolas, P. (2022). Imagining non-carceral futures with(in) Mad Studies. In P. Beresford & J. Russo (Eds.), *The Routledge international handbook of Mad Studies* (pp. 217–222). Routledge. https://doi.org/10.4324/9780429465444-27

Kaufman-Mthimkhulu, S. L. (2020, June 6). *We don't need cops to become social workers: We need peer support + community response networks*. Medium. https://medium.

com/@stefkaufman/we-dont-need-cops-to-become-social-workers-we-need-peer-support-b8e6c4ffe87a

Kanani, N. & Pilling, M. D. (2014, May 24–30). *The student mental health crisis? Managing structural violence and student wellbeing through university mental health strategies* [Conference presentation]. Congress of the Humanities and Social Sciences, St Catharines, ON.

Kilty, J. (2018). Carceral optics and the crucible of segregation: Revising scenes of state-sanctioned violence against incarcerated women. In J. Kilty & E. Dej (Eds.), *Containing madness: Gender and "psy" in institutional contexts* (pp. 119–144). Palgrave Macmillan. https://doi.org/10.1007/978-3-319-89749-3_6

Kilty, J. M. & Lehalle, S. (2019). Mad, bad, and stuck in the hole: Carceral segregation as slow violence. In A. Daley, L. Costa, & P. Beresford (Eds.), *Madness, violence and power: A critical collection* (pp. 310–329). University of Toronto Press. https://doi.org/10.3138/9781442629981-026

Kilty, J. M. & Orsini, M. (2024). Emotions and anti-carceral advocacy in Canada: "All of the anger this creates in our bodies is also a tool to kill us". *Policy & Politics, 52*(2), 219–238. https://doi.org/10.1332/03055736y2023d000000024

Kinitz, D. J., Goodyear, T., Dromer, E., Gesink, D., Ferlatte, O., Knight, R., & Salway, T. (2022). "Conversion therapy" experiences in their social contexts: A qualitative study of sexual orientation and gender identity and expression change efforts in Canada. *The Canadian Journal of Psychiatry, 67*(6), 441–451. https://doi.org/10.1177/07067437211030498

Krazinski, M., Cosantino, J., Poole, J., & Friedman, M. (2023). *Maddening the Academy Call for Abstracts*. International Mad Studies Journal. https://docs.google.com/document/d/e/2PACX-1vTlHcfa54_hj9tEbB8fh8L_237sJ__vkY4Wu4dFifV_rzvut5nSIs1CZs2wkGUjC_XTb7-B-P5k6AIs/pub?fbclid=IwAR1LRfYqFF5gdoOsh_037BvFYFqYav4pbx2_5Z_NXbrYdEUoB5yNam9tJP0

Landry, D. & Church, K. (2016). Teaching (like) crazy in a mad positive school: Exploring the charms of recursion.

In J. Russo & A. Sweeney (Eds.), *Searching for a rose garden: Challenging psychiatry, fostering Mad Studies* (pp. 172–182). PCCS Books.

Landry, D. (2017). Survivor research in Canada: "Talking" recovery, resisting psychiatry, and reclaiming madness. *Disability & Society, 32*(9), 1437–1457. https://doi.org/10.32920/14639283

Lee-Evoy, J. (2019). Institutional Oppression and Violence as Self-Defence. In A. Daley, L. Costa, & P. Beresford (Eds.), *Madness, violence and power: A critical collection* (pp. 286–294). University of Toronto Press. https://doi.org/10.3138/9781442629981-024

LeFrançois, B. A. & Voronka, J. (2022). Mad epistemologies and maddening the ethics of knowledge production. In T. Macías (Ed.), *Unravelling research: The ethics and politics of research in the social sciences* (pp. 105–130). Fernwood Publishing.

Levine, B. (2024, June 6). *How to explain top psychiatrists' "Dr. Strangelove exuberance" unchecked by reality.* Mad in America. www.madinamerica.com/2024/06/how-to-explain-top-psychiatrists-dr-strangelove-exuberance-unchecked-by-reality/

Library Company of Philadelphia. (n.d.). *Hearing voices: Memoirs from the margins of mental health.* https://library-company.org/hearingvoices-online/index.html

Logan, J. & Karter, J. M. (2022). Psychiatrization of resistance: The co-option of consumer, survivor, and ex-patient movements in the global south. *Frontiers in Sociology, 7*(784390). https://doi.org/10.3389/fsoc.2022.784390

Lovell-Norton, J., Poursanidou, K., Machin, K., Jeffreys, S., & Dale, H. (2021). How can we survive and thrive as survivor researchers? In H. McLaughlin, P. Beresford, C. Cameron, H. Casey, & J. Duffy, *The Routledge handbook of service user involvement in human services research and education* (pp. 403–418). Routledge. https://doi.org/10.4324/9780429433306-42

Macintosh, J. (2023). Ode to the MSc in Mad Studies. *Asylum, 30*(4), 6–7.

MacKinnon, K. R., Guta, A., Voronka, J., Pilling, M., Williams, C. C., Strike, C., & Ross, L. E. (2021). The political economy of peer research: mapping the possibilities and precarities of paying people for lived experience. *The British Journal of Social Work*, *51*(3), 888–906. https://doi.org/10.1093/bjsw/bcaa241

Mad Student Zine Team. (2022a). Origins of Outliers. In Mad Student Zine Team (Eds.), *Outliers: Teaching & learning beyond the norms* [Zine] 2. MacPherson Institute, McMaster University. http://hdl.handle.net/11375/27906

Mad Student Zine Team. (2022b). *Outliers: Teaching & learning beyond the norms* [Zine] 2. MacPherson Institute, McMaster University. http://hdl.handle.net/11375/27906

Mariette, S. (2024). Surveillance is not "safety." *Asylum*, *31*(1), 12–13.

Maylea, C. & Daya, I. (2019, October 19). *When Mad voices are locked out of academia.* Mad In America. www.madinamerica.com/2019/10/mad-voices-locked-out-academia/

McCreary, T. & Hall, R. (2024). The healer, the witch, and the law: The settler magic that criminalized Indigenous medicine men as frauds and normalized colonial violence as care. *Annals of the American Association of Geographers*, *114*(2), 352–368. https://doi.org/10.1080/24694452.2023.2267152

McEwen, D. (2022). *Mad futures now: Avant-garde dishumanism in the poetry of Claude Gauvreau, Hannah Weiner, and bill bissett* [Doctoral dissertation, Brock University]. Brock Theses.

McKeown, M., Scholes, A., Jones, F., & Aindow, W. (2019). Coercive practices in mental health services: stories of recalcitrance, resistance and legitimation. In A. Daley, L. Costa, & P. Beresford (Eds.), *Madness, violence and power: A critical collection* (pp. 263–285). University of Toronto Press. https://doi.org/10.3138/9781442629981-023

McRuer, R. (2006). Compulsory able-bodiedness and queer/disabled existence. In L. J. David (Ed.), *The disability studies reader* (2nd ed.) (pp. 301–308). Routledge. https://doi.org/10.4324/9780203077887-37

Menzies, R. & Palys, T. (2006). Turbulent spirits: Aboriginal patients in the British Columbia psychiatric system, 1879–1950. In J. E. Moran & D. Wright (Eds.), *Mental health and Canadian society: Historical perspectives* (pp. 149–175). McGill-Queen's University Press. https://doi.org/10.1515/9780773576544-010

Minkowitz, T. (2010). Abolishing mental health laws to comply with the Convention on the Rights of Persons with Disabilities. In B. McSherry & P. Weller (Eds.), *Rethinking rights-based mental health laws* (pp. 151–177). Hart Publishing. https://doi.org/10.5040/9781474200714.ch-007

Mosher, L. & Cohen, D. (2003). The ethics of electroconvulsive therapy. *Virtual Mentor: American Medical Association Journal of Ethics, 5*(1), 463–466. https://doi.org/10.1001/virtualmentor.2003.5.10.oped1-0310

Netchitailova, E. (2019). The mystery of madness through art and Mad Studies. *Disability & Society, 34*(9–10), 1509–1515. https://doi.org/10.1080/09687599.2019.1619236

Neil, C. (2021, June 20). *Appeal to Board of Health to ban ECT in Ontario.* Mad in Canada. https://madincanada.org/2021/06/appeal-to-board-of-health-to-ban-ect-in-ontario/

Neilson, S., Chittle, A., & Zaheer, J. (2019). Handcuffed: Rethinking physical restraints for mental health transfers in university settings. *Canadian Family Physician, 65*(7), 460–462. https://doi.org/10.9778/cmajo.20210135

Newman, J., Boxall, K., Jury, R., & Dickinson, J. (2022). Professional education and Mad Studies: learning and teaching about service users' understandings of mental and emotional distress. *Disability & Society, 34*(9–10), 1523–1547. https://doi.org/10.1080/09687599.2019.1594697

Norvoll, R. & Pedersen, R. (2016). Exploring the views of people with mental health problems on the concept of coercion: Towards a broader socio-ethical perspective. *Social Science & Medicine, 156*, 204–211.

Ormerod, E., Beresford, P., Carr, S., Gould, D., Jeffreys, S., Machin, K., Poursanidou, D., Thompson, S., & Yiannoullou, S. (2018). *SRN Manifesto.* Survivor Researcher Network.

https://survivorresearcher.net/wp-content/uploads/2021/04/2018_SRN_MANIFESTO.pdf

Papoulias, S. (C). & Callard, F. (2021). "A limpet on a ship": Spatio-temporal dynamics of patient and public involvement in research. *Health Expectations*, *24*(2), 810–818. https://doi.org/10.1111/hex.13215

Papoulias, S. (C). & Callard, F. (2022). Material and epistemic precarity: It's time to talk about labour exploitation in mental health research. *Social Science & Medicine*, *306*(115102). https://doi.org/10.1016/j.socscimed.2022.115102

Persaud, S., Myer, J., Shanouda, F., Pilling, M. D., Pitt, K. A., Voronka, J., & Ross, L. (2024, June 12–21). *Mapping the 'wellness complex': Examining graduate student mental health through a critical disability studies lens* [Conference presentation]. Congress of the Humanities and Social Sciences, Montreal, QC.

Persaud, S. (2022). *No sovereign remedy: Distress, madness, and mental health care in Guyana* [Doctoral dissertation, York University]. YorkSpace.

Pickens, T. A. (2019). *Black madness: Mad Blackness*. Duke University Press. https://doi.org/10.1515/9781478005506

Pilling, M. D. (2022). *Queer and trans madness: Struggles for social justice*. Palgrave Macmillan. https://doi.org/10.1007/978-3-030-90413-5

Pilling, M. D. (Forthcoming). Toward mad trans liberation: The necessity of a mad-queer-trans lens. In B. LeFrançois, I. Abdillahi, G. Reaume, & R. Menzies (Eds.), *Mad matters: A critical reader in Canadian Mad Studies* (2nd ed.). Canadian Scholars Press.

Pilling, M. D., Daley, A., Gibson, M. F., Ross, L. E., & Zaheer, J. (2018). Assessing "insight," determining agency and autonomy: Implicating social identities. In J. Kilty & E. Dej (Eds.), *Containing madness: Gender and "psy" in institutional contexts* (pp. 191–213). Palgrave Macmillan. https://doi.org/10.1007/978-3-319-89749-3_9

Poole, J. M. & Grant, Z. S. (2018). When youth get mad through a critical course on mental health. In S. Pashang,

N. Khanlou, & J. Clarke (Eds.), *Today's youth and mental health: Hope, power, and resilience* (pp. 305–320). Springer Cham. https://doi.org/10.1007/978-3-319-64838-5_17

Price, M. (2011). *Mad at school: Rhetorics of mental disability and academic life.* University of Michigan Press. https://doi.org/10.3998/mpub.1612837

Price, M. (2015). The bodymind problem and the possibilities of pain. *Hypatia, 30*(1), 268–284. https://doi.org/10.1111/hypa.12127

Reaume, G. (2006). Mad people's history. *Radical History Review, 2006*(94), 170–182. https://doi.org/10.1215/01636545-2006-94-170

Reaume, G. (2008). A history of lobotomy in Ontario. In E. A. Heaman, A. Li, and S. McKellar (Eds.), *Essays in honour of Michael Bliss: Figuring the social* (pp. 378–399). University of Toronto Press. https://doi.org/10.3138/9781442688025-019

Reaume, G. (2019). Creating Mad People's History as a university credit course since 2000. *New Horizons in Adult Education and Human Resource Development, 31*(1), 22–39. https://doi.org/10.1002/nha3.20238

Reaume, G. (2024). The qualitative historical origins of Mad Studies in word and deed, 1436–1914. *Qualitative Inquiry.* https://doi.org/10.1177/10778004241253249

Read, J. (2023, November 17). *Is it time to ban electroconvulsive therapy on children?* Psychology Today. 'www.psychologytoday.com/intl/blog/psychiatry-through-the-looking-glass/202311/is-it-time-to-ban-electroconvulsive-therapy-for#:~:text=ECT%20has%20been%20banned%20altogether,on%20children%20is%20not%20prohibited.

Recovery in the Bin. (2018, July). *A Simple Guide to Co-Production.* https://recoveryinthebin.org/a-simple-guide-to-co-production/

Reel, K. (2019) "Gravity and grace": Acknowledging restraint and seclusion as a violence. In A. Daley, L. Costa, & P. Beresford (Eds.), *Madness, violence and power: A critical collection* (pp. 295–309). University of Toronto Press. https://doi.org/10.3138/9781442629981-025

Reid, J. (2018, July 17). *Asking questions about mental health in the arts*. Canadian Art. https://canadianart.ca/features/workman-arts-bigfeels-symposium/

Reid, J. (2019). *Materializing a mad aesthetic through the making of politicized fibre art* [Doctoral dissertation, York University]. YorkSpace.

Reid, J., & Poole, J. (2013). Mad students in the social work classroom? Notes from the beginnings of an inquiry. *Journal of Progressive Human Services*, 24(3), 209–222. https://doi.org/10.1080/10428232.2013.835185

Reid, J., Snyder, S. N., Voronka, J., Landry, D., & Church, K. (2019). Mobilizing Mad art in the neoliberal university: Resisting regulatory efforts by inscribing art as political practice. *Journal of Literary & Cultural Disability Studies*, 13(3), 255–271. https://doi.org/10.3828/jlcds.2019.20

Rembis, M. (2014). The new asylums: Madness and mass incarceration in the neoliberal era. In L. Ben-Mosche (Ed.), *Disability incarcerated: Imprisonment and disability in the United States and Canada* (pp. 139–159). Palgrave Macmillan. https://doi.org/10.1057/9781137388476_8

Reville, D. (2013). Is Mad Studies emerging as a new field of inquiry? In B. A. LeFrançois, R. Menzies, & G. Reaume, *Mad matters: A critical reader in Canadian Mad Studies* (pp. 170–180). Canadian Scholars Press.

Reville, D. (2022). Taking Mad Studies back out into the community. In P. Beresford & J. Russo (Eds.), *The Routledge international handbook of Mad Studies* (pp. 307–314). Routledge. https://doi.org/10.4324/9780429465444-36

Reville, D. & Church, K. (2012). Mad activism enters its fifth decade: Psychiatric survivor organizing in Toronto. In A. Choudry, J. Hanley, & E. Shragge (Eds.), *Organize! Building from the local for global justice* (pp. 189–201). PM Press.

Rice, C., Dion, S. D., & Chandler, E. (2021). Decolonizing disability through activist art. *Disability Studies Quarterly*, 41(2). https://doi.org/10.18061/dsq.v41i2.7130

Rivest, M. P. (2022). When lay knowledge is a symptom: The uses of insight in psychiatric interventions. *Studies in*

Social Justice, 16(1), 245–263. https://doi.org/10.26522/ssj. v16i1.2681

Rodéhn, C. (2022). Introducing Mad Studies and Mad reading to Game Studies. *Game Studies, 22*(1).

Roman, L. G., Brown, S., Noble, S., Wainer, R., & Young, A. E. (2009). No time for nostalgia!: Asylum-making, medicalized colonialism in British Columbia (1859–97) and artistic praxis for social transformation. *International Journal of Qualitative Studies in Education, 22*(1), 17–63. https://doi. org/10.1080/09518390802581919

Roper, C. & Gooding, P. (2018). This is not a story: From ethical loneliness to respect for diverse ways of knowing, thinking and being. In E. Flynn, A. Arstein-Kerslake, C. D. Bhailís, & M. L. Serra (Eds.), *Global perspectives on legal capacity reform* (pp. 154–164). Routledge. https://doi. org/10.4324/9781315098302-20

Roquemore, K. & Cosantino, J. (2024, April 24–26). *MadTransCrip pedagogies and pedagogical lifeworlds: An exploration.* [Conference presentation]. New England Educational Research Organization, Portsmouth, NH.

Rose, D. (2001). Users' voices: The perspectives of mental health service users on community and hospital care. *Psychiatric Bulletin, 26*(3), 118–119. https://doi.org/10.1192/ pb.26.3.118-b

Rose, D. (2022). *Mad knowledges and user-led research.* Palgrave Macmillan. https://doi.org/10.1007/978-3-031-07551-3

Rose, D. (2023). Is there power in Mad knowledge? *Social Theory & Health, 21*(4), 305–319. https://doi.org/10.1057/ s41285-023-00194-y

Rose, D. & Beresford, P. (2024). PPI in psychiatry and the problem of knowledge. *BMC Psychiatry, 24*(1), 52. https:// doi.org/10.1186/s12888-023-05398-0

Rose, D., Carr, S., & Beresford, P. (2018). 'Widening crossdisciplinary research for mental health': What is missing from the Research Councils UK mental health agenda? *Disability & Society, 33*(3), 476–481. https://doi.org/10.1080/09687599. 2018.1423907

Rose, D. & Kalathil, J. (2019). Power, privilege and knowledge: The untenable promise of co-production in mental "health." *Frontiers in Sociology, 4.* https://doi.org/10.3389/fsoc.2019.00057

Ross, L. & Pilling, M.D. (2024, January 25). *Ethical tensions and harms in peer research and engagement* [Webinar]. Evidence Exchange Network.

Ross, L. E., Pilling, M., Voronka, J., Pitt, K. A., McLean, E., King, C., Shakya, Y., MacKinnon, K. R., Williams, C., Strike, C., & Guta, A. (2023). "I will play this tokenistic game, I just want something useful for my community": Experiences of and resistance to harms of peer research. *Critical Public Health, 33*(5), 735–746. https://doi.org/10.1080/09581596.2023.2268822

Russo, J. (2023). Psychiatrization, assertions of epistemic justice, and the question of agency. *Frontiers in Sociology, 8*(1092298). https://doi.org/10.3389/fsoc.2023.1092298

Russo, J. (2012). Survivor-controlled research: A new foundation for thinking about psychiatry and mental health. *Forum Qualitative Sozialforschung/Forum: Qualitative Social Research, 13*(1). https://doi.org/10.17169/fqs-13.1.1790

Salway, T. & Ashley, F. (2022). Ridding Canadian medicine of conversion therapy. *Canadian Medical Association Journal, 194*(1), E17–E18. https://doi.org/10.1503/cmaj.211709

Saisi, B. (2021). Barred by the maddening state: Mental health and incarceration in the heterosexist, anti-Black, settler colonial carceral state. In M. J. Coyle & D. Scott (Eds.), *The Routledge international handbook of penal abolition* (pp. 217–228). Routledge. https://doi.org/10.4324/9780429425035-34

Sampson, A., Cowley, J., Szeto, E., & Tomlinson, A. (2022, March 27). *Conversion therapy is illegal in Canada. But some U.S. life coaches are offering it to Canadians online.* CBC News. www.cbc.ca/news/canada/marketplace-life-coachconversion-therapy-1.6369104

Scott, A. & Doughty, C. (2012). Care, empowerment and self-determination in the practice of peer support. *Disability*

& Society, 27(7), 1011–1024. https://doi.org/10.1080/09687599.2012.695578

Shanouda, F. (2023). Fat and mad bodies: Out of, under, and beyond control. In A. Taylor, K. Ioannoni, R. A. Bahra, C. Evans, A. Scrivener, & M. Fieldman (Eds.), *Fat studies in Canada:(Re) Mapping the field* (pp. 355–372). Inanna Publications.

Sharma, P. (2023). *Barriers to recovery from 'psychosis': A peer investigation of psychiatric subjectivation*. Routledge. https://doi.org/10.4324/9781003248804

Shaw, F. (2022, July 11). *Human rights laws needed to end coercive psychiatric practices against African Americans*. CCR International's Task Force Against Racism & Modern Day Eugenics. www.cchrtaskforce.org/post/end-coercive-psychiatric-practices-against-african-americans

Sheldon, C. T. & Spector, K. R. (2019). Law as a site of Mad resistance: User and refuser perspectives in legal challenges to psychiatric detention. *Journal of Ethics in Mental Health*, 10.

Shephard, M., Ellenwood, L., & Oke, C. (2020, Oct 21). *Brainwashed: The echoes of MK-ULTRA*. CBC News. https://newsinteractives.cbc.ca/longform/brainwashed-mkultra/

Snyder, S. N., Pitt, K. A., Shanouda, F., Voronka, J., Reid, J., & Landry, D. (2019). Unlearning through Mad Studies: Disruptive pedagogical praxis. *Curriculum Inquiry*, 49(4), 485–502. https://doi.org/10.1080/03626784.2019.1664254

Spandler, H. & Barker M. J. (2016, 1 July). *Mad and Queer Studies: Interconnections and tensions*. Mad Studies Network. https://madstudies2014.wordpress.com/2016/07/01/mad-and-queer-studies-interconnections-and-tensions/

Spandler, H. & Poursanidou, D. (2019). Who is included in the Mad Studies project? *The Journal of Ethics in Mental Health*, 10.

Steele, L. (2017). Disabling forensic mental health detention: The carcerality of the disabled body. *Punishment & Society*, 19(3), 327–347. https://doi.org/10.1177/1462474516680204

Swain, G. (2019). The healing power of art in intergenerational trauma: Race, sex, age and disability. *Canadian Journal of Disability Studies*, 8(1), 15–31. https://doi.org/10.15353/cjds.v8i1.469

Sweeney, A. (2016). Why Mad Studies needs survivor research and survivor research needs Mad Studies. *Intersectionalities: A Global Journal of Social Work Analysis, Research, Polity, and Practice*, 5(3), 36–61.

Thorneycroft, R. (2020). Crip theory and Mad Studies: Intersections and points of departure. *Canadian Journal of Disability Studies*, 9(1), 91–121. https://doi.org/10.15353/cjds. v9i1.597

Timander, A. (2020). Involuntary care and treatment in psychiatric settings – Manifestations of power and violence? *Scandinavian Journal of Disability Research*, 22(1), 351–359. https://doi.org/10.16993/sjdr.684

Trans Lifeline (2020). Why no nonconsensual active rescue? In E. Dixon & L. L. Piepzna-Samarasinha (Eds.), *Beyond survival: Strategies and stories from the transformative justice movement* (pp. 135–140). AK Press.

Tseris, E. J., Bright Hart, E., & Franks, S. (2022). "My voice was discounted the whole way through": A gendered analysis of women's experiences of involuntary mental health treatment. *Affilia*, 37(4), 645–663. https://doi.org/10.1177/08861099221108714

Trivedi, P. (2008). Black service user involvement: Rhetoric or reality? in S. Fernando and F. Keating (Eds.), *Mental health in a multi-ethnic society* (2nd ed.) (pp.136–146). Routledge. https://doi.org/10.4324/9780203895535

Turner, M. & Beresford, P. (2005). *User controlled research: Its meaning and potential. Final Report.* Shaping Our Lives/ Brunel University Centre for Citizen Participation. https:// shapingourlives.org.uk/report/user-controlled-research-its-meanings-and-potential/

van Daalen-Smith, C., Adam, S., Breggin, P., & LeFrançois, B. A. (2014). The utmost discretion: How presumed prudence leaves children susceptible to electroshock. *Children & Society*, 28(3), 205–217. https://doi.org/10.1111/chso.12073

van Daalen-Smith, C. L. (2011). Waiting for oblivion: Women's experiences with electroshock. *Issues in Mental Health Nursing*, 32, 457–472. https://doi.org/10.3109/01612840. 2011.583810 van Daalen-Smith, C., Hagen, B., & Breggin, P. (2015). Diminished: Canadian women's experiences of electroshock. *Atlantis: Critical Studies in Gender, Culture & Social Justice*, 37(1), 143–155.

Voronka, J. (2016). The politics of "people with lived experience": Experiential authority and the risks of strategic essentialism. *Philosophy, Psychiatry, & Psychology*, 23(3), 189–201. https://doi.org/10.1353/ppp.2016.0017

Voronka, J. (2017). Turning mad knowledge into affective labor: The case of the peer support worker. *American Quarterly*, 69(2), 333–338. https://doi.org/10.1353/aq.2017.0029

Voronka, J. (2019). The mental health peer worker as inform-ant: Performing authenticity and the paradoxes of passing. *Disability & Society*, 34(4), 564–582. https://doi.org/10.10 80/09687599.2018.1545113

Voronka, J. & King, C. (2023). Reflections on peer research: Powers, pleasures, pains. *The British Journal of Social Work*, 53(3), 1692–1699. https://doi.org/10.1093/bjsw/bcad010

Walker, D. (2015, March 14). *Horse-stealing mania: The Hiawatha Asylum for Insane Indians*. Mad in America. www.madinamerica.com/2015/03/horse-stealing-mania-hiawatha-asylum-insane-indians/

Walker, D. E. (2022). *Coyote's swing: A memoir and critique of mental hygiene in Native America*. Washington State University Press.

Walter, L. (2022, November 25). *Mad art and the contested mind*. Mentoring Artists for Women's Art. https://mawa.ca/newsletters/critical-writing/mad-art-and-the-contested-mind

Weitz, D. (1988). Notes of a "schizophrenic" shitdisturber. In B. Burstow & D. Weitz (Eds.), *Shrink resistant* (pp. 285–302). New Star Books.

Weitz, D. (2013). Eletroshock: Torture as "treatment." In B. A. LeFrançois, R. Menzies, & G. Reaume, *Mad matters: A critical reader in Canadian Mad Studies* (pp. 158–169). Canadian Scholars Press.

Weitz, D. (2018). *Resistance matters: The radical vision of an antipsychiatry activist*. Mad in America. www.madinamerica.com/wp-content/uploads/2019/06/Resistance-Matters-April-2019.pdf

Whitt, S. (2021). "Care and maintenance": Indigeneity, disability and settler colonialism at the Canton Asylum for Insane Indians, 1902–1934. *Disability Studies Quarterly*, *41*(4). https://doi.org/10.18061/dsq.v41i4.8463

Whitaker, R. (2002). *Mad in America: Bad science, bad medicine, and the enduring mistreatment of the mentally ill.* Basic Books.

Wipond, R. (2023, November 17). Crisis hotlines, like Canada's new 988, promise confidentiality. So why do so many trace calls and texts? *The Globe and Mail.* www.theglobeandmail.com/opinion/article-crisis-hotlines-like-canadas-new-988-promise-confidentiality-so-why-do/

Wipond, R. (2024). *Your consent is not required: The rise in psychiatric detentions, forced treatment, and abusive guardianships.* BenBella Books.

Wolframe, P. (2012). The madwoman in the academy, or, revealing the invisible straightjacket: Theorizing and teaching saneism and sane privilege. *Disability Studies Quarterly*, *33*(1). https://doi.org/10.18061/dsq.v33i1.3425

Wolframe, P. (2014). *Reading through madness: Counter-psychiatric epistemologies and the biopolitics of (in)sanity in post-World War II Anglo Atlantic women's narratives* (Publication No. 8733 9760 4947689) [Doctoral dissertation, McMaster University]. MacSphere Open Access Dissertations and Theses.

Wright, B. A. (1990). An historical review of electroconvulsive therapy. *Jefferson Journal of Psychiatry*, *8*(2), 68–74. https://doi.org/10.29046/JJP.008.2.007

Yellow Bird, P. (2004). *Wild Indians: Native perspectives on the Hiawatha Asylum for Insane Indians.* National Empowerment Center. https://power2u.org/wp-content/uploads/2017/01/NativePerspectivesPeminaYellowBird.pdf

Zaheer, J. (2021). Documenting restraint: Minimizing trauma. In A. Daley & M. D. Pilling (Eds.), *Interrogating psychiatric narratives of madness: Documented lives* (pp. 111–135). Palgrave Macmillan. https://doi.org/10.1007/978-3-030-83692-4_5

INDEX

Note: Page numbers followed by "n" denote endnotes.

For Product Safety Concerns and Information please contact our EU
representative GPSR@taylorandfrancis.com
Taylor & Francis Verlag GmbH, Kaufingerstraße 24, 80331 München, Germany

www.ingramcontent.com/pod-product-compliance
Lightning Source LLC
Chambersburg PA
CBHW071104280326
41928CB00051B/2807